Human Factors in Surgery

Tara N. Cohen • Eric J. Ley
Bruce L. Gewertz
Editors

Human Factors in Surgery

Enhancing Safety and Flow in Patient Care

Springer

Editors
Tara N. Cohen
Cedars-Sinai Medical Center
Los Angeles, CA
USA

Eric J. Ley
Cedars-Sinai Medical Center
Los Angeles, CA
USA

Bruce L. Gewertz
Cedars-Sinai Medical Center
Los Angeles, CA
USA

ISBN 978-3-030-53126-3 ISBN 978-3-030-53127-0 (eBook)
https://doi.org/10.1007/978-3-030-53127-0

This Springer imprint is published by the registered company Springer Nature Switzerland AG
The registered company address is: Gewerbestrasse 11, 6330 Cham, Switzerland

"To our colleagues who selflessly take superb care of patients and make that care safer"

Foreword

Sarah slumped into a chair. "I'm cooked," she said in a halting voice. A talented surgeon devoted to her patients and to safe surgery, Sarah had performed a "wrong site surgery." It was her second.

Today's story was easy to piece together. She had four cases scheduled and they proceeded in a manner not unfamiliar to any surgeon. A cholecystectomy had been straightforward until, just as a little bit of bleeding had started, the insufflation failed. Unable to see, Sarah asked that the circulator change the CO2 bottle. The circulator was from another room—the regular circulator was on break. Everybody watched with impatience as the circulator fumbled with the valve. Sarah said, "Yes, in retrospect, I got agitated."

While this case was delayed waiting for help, another force was at work nearby. The two following cases were breast operations. One was a lumpectomy and sentinel node biopsy for breast cancer. So was the case after that. Because one patient had eaten recently, the order of the cases was switched.

"The nurse read the timeout in the usual manner," Sarah told me. "I was still worked up from the previous case and depended on the team for the checklist. I may have been told about the switch, but I don't remember it. I made a mistake."

This story illustrates why this book is so important to any practitioner of medicine but especially to anyone who holds a sharp knife in her hand. As surgeons interface with systems and machines, we must know how human factors can help mitigate the risks that face our patients and us.

Sarah knew that she would be reprimanded and fined by the state board of medicine and that a malpractice suit would be likely. At the sharp end of the stick, she would be held responsible for the mistake. In most other worlds, a system analysis would uncover the several causes of the mistake. They include the institution' system of allowing untrained circulators to substitute for others, the inaccurate and largely lip service way in which timeouts were conducted, the pressure to utilize OR time efficiently, the added risk when laterality is considered, and a culture of deference to surgeons, among others. Additionally, the interface with CO2 tanks, cameras, and complex equipment would be examined. Why do we "run out of gas" so often?

In the pages that follow, you will learn how to protect yourself and your patients from what can be chaotic systems. If you are in a position of administration, you will see how blaming the surgeon is misguided. You will start to see how systems and equipment interact with human beings, fallible human beings, and how those systems often leave hard working practitioners hanging out there on their own.

You will learn, again, that no surgeon wakens in the morning with the intent of harming a patient.

Tampa, FL, USA

Richard Karl

Acknowledgments

The editors wish to acknowledge the remarkable mentorship they received during their training and early careers. Tara was strongly influenced by Christy Helgeson, Scott Shappell, Douglas Wiegmann, and Susan Hallbeck who have worked tirelessly to optimize safety and well-being across several industries and have guided and encouraged her to do the same. Eric would like to specifically recognize Gerald Westheimer, Ed Ray, Robert Beart, and Demetrios Demetriades for their insights and encouragement at various stages of his career. Bruce will never forget the professionalism of Herb Cohn, Tom Dent, Jim Stanley, and Bill Fry who cared about their patients above all and took the time to teach him the same.

About the Book

Human Factors in Surgery: Enhancing Safety and Flow in Patient Care delivers a comprehensive review of human factors principles as they relate to the operating theatre. Hippocrates was the first to suggest the environment, lighting, and instrumentation used can impact surgical performance. Throughout history, the science of human factors has advanced with aviation due to a combination of engineering, management science, and applied psychological research. Human factors research is a key component of modern safety and performance improvement in high-risk industries including road and rail transport, aviation, shipping, mining, nuclear power, and the military. Despite this, surgical care has been late to adopt human factors principles. The traditional belief suggests life or death depends largely on the technical ability of the skilled surgeon. However, research across the globe has demonstrated the organization and operation of a given system can also contribute to surgical outcomes. *Human Factors in Surgery: Enhancing Safety and Flow in Patient Care* provides examples of how appropriately designed systems can lead to success where previously there was failure. The implementation of effective human factors principles may be lifesaving.

The textbook provides multidimensional human-centered insights from the viewpoint of academic surgeons and experts in human factors engineering to improve workflow, treatment time, and outcomes. This text provides an overview of human factors as it relates to the operating theatre. The authors (consisting of both surgeons and human factors experts) focus on describing elements of the surgical system and highlighting the lessons learned from systems engineering. The developers aimed to create a handbook that all surgeons at any level in their training could read to improve their practice. To guide the reader, the book will begin broadly with Human Factors Principles for Surgery then narrow to a discussion of broad surgical considerations followed by insights regarding specific surgical areas. The early human factors chapters are written by experts in human factors and focus on describing methods used to study and improve interacting systemic factors in surgery. The chapters focused on specific surgical specialties and scenarios are written by experienced surgeons who have inherently adapted the principles of human factors to facilitate the care of their patients. Each chapter follows the following structure: (1) an overview of the topic at hand to provide a reference for readers, (2) a case study or story to illustrate the topic, (3) a discussion of the topic including human factors insights, and (4) lessons learned or personal "pearls" related to improving the specific system described.

Contents

Editors and Contributors

About the Editors

Tara N. Cohen, PhD, is the Director of Surgical Safety and Human Factors Research at Cedars-Sinai Medical Center. Tara earned her Doctorate in Human Factors from Embry-Riddle Aeronautical University. Her primary research interests involve applying human factors methodologies to identify opportunities to improve safety, efficiency and well-being in healthcare. Most recently, her work has focused on utilizing observational research methods to identify and mitigate barriers to surgical system safety and flow.

Eric J. Ley, MD, is the Director of the Surgical Intensive Care Unit and Program Director for the Trauma and Critical Care Fellowship and has worked on multiple projects that utilize human factors to improve the delivery of trauma and intensive unit care. Dr. Ley has redesigned patient flow from the trauma bay to the operating room by reducing flow disruptions.

Bruce L. Gewertz, MD, is Surgeon-in-Chief, Chair of the Department of Surgery, Vice President for Interventional Services, and Vice Dean of Academic Affairs at Cedars-Sinai. He also holds the H & S Nichols Distinguished Chair in Surgery. Dr. Gewertz is the author of more than 250 original articles, book chapters, and books. His principal clinical interests include cerebrovascular disease and physician leadership skills. The National Institutes of Health and the American Heart Association have funded his basic research into cellular mechanisms of ischemia-reperfusion injury. Recently, he was the principal investigator of a $4.4 million project funded by the Department of Defense on the optimization of human factors in civilian and military operating rooms.

Contributors

James H. Abernathy, MD Department of Anesthesiology and Critical Care Medicine, Johns Hopkins University, Baltimore, MD, USA

Myrtede C. Alfred, PhD Clinical Human Factors and Applied Safety Science Unit, Department of Anesthesia and Perioperative Medicine, Medical University of South Carolina, Charleston, SC, USA

Jennifer T. Anger, MD Department of Surgery, Division of Urology, Cedars-Sinai Medical Center, Los Angeles, CA, USA

Ali Azizzadeh, MD Department of Surgery, Division of Vascular Surgery, Cedars-Sinai Medical Center, Los Angeles, CA, USA

David Bliss, MD Pediatric Surgery, Cedars-Sinai Medical Center, Los Angeles, CA, USA

Ken R. Catchpole, PhD Clinical Human Factors and Applied Safety Science Unit, Department of Anesthesia and Perioperative Medicine, Medical University of South Carolina, Charleston, SC, USA

Barbara S. Chaparro, PhD Department of Human Factors and Behavioral Neurobiology, Embry-Riddle Aeronautical University, Daytona Beach, FL, USA

Kate Cohen, MS Department of Surgery, Cedars-Sinai Medical Center, Los Angeles, CA, USA

Tara N. Cohen, PhD Department of Surgery, Cedars-Sinai Medical Center, Los Angeles, CA, USA

Jessica S. Crystal, MD Surgical Oncology, Cedars-Sinai Medical Center, Los Angeles, CA, USA

Anahat Dhillon, MD Department of Anesthesiology, Cedars-Sinai Medical Center, Los Angeles, CA, USA

Justin B. Dimick, MD Department of Surgery, Michigan Medicine, Ann Arbor, MI, USA

Ashley Fejleh, DO Department of Anesthesiology, Cedars-Sinai Medical Center, Los Angeles, CA, USA

Phillip R. Fleshner, MD Cedars-Sinai Medical Center, Los Angeles, CA, USA

Paul Frank, MD Department of Anesthesiology, Cedars-Sinai Medical Center, Los Angeles, CA, USA

Alexandra Gangi, MD Surgical Oncology, Cedars-Sinai Medical Center, Los Angeles, CA, USA

Bruce L. Gewertz, MD Department of Surgery, Cedars-Sinai Medical Center, Los Angeles, CA, USA

Caprice C. Greenberg, MD Department of Surgery, University of Wisconsin School of Medicine and Public Health, Madison, WI, USA

Andrew C. Griggs, MS Department of Human Factors and Behavioral Neurobiology, Embry-Riddle Aeronautical University, Daytona Beach, FL, USA

Jake F. Hemingway, MD PGY-4 Integrated Vascular Surgery, University of Washington, Seattle, WA, USA

Monica Jain, MD Department of Surgery, Cedars-Sinai Medical Center, Los Angeles, CA, USA

Falisha F. Kanji, BA Department of Surgery, Cedars-Sinai Medical Center, Los Angeles, CA, USA

Irene Kim, MD Comprehensive Transplant Center, Department of Surgery, Cedars-Sinai Medical Center, Los Angeles, CA, USA

Mehreen Kisat, MD Brigham and Women's Hospital, Boston, MA, USA

Elizabeth H. Lazzara, PhD Department of Human Factors and Behavioral Neurobiology, Embry-Riddle Aeronautical University, Daytona Beach, FL, USA

Jessica Lee, MD Critical Care Medicine Anesthesiology, Cedars-Sinai Medical Center, Los Angeles, CA, USA

Tiffany Leverenz, PhD Human Factors Engineer, Intuitive Surgical, Sunnyvale, CA, USA

Eric J. Ley, MD Department of Surgery, Cedars-Sinai Medical Center, Los Angeles, CA, USA

Douglas Z. Liou, MD Division of Thoracic Surgery, Department of Cardiothoracic Surgery, Stanford University, Stanford, CA, USA

Bethany Lowndes, PhD Department of Neurological Sciences, University of Nebraska Medical Center, Omaha, NE, USA

Matthew J. Martin, MD Trauma and Emergency Surgery Service, Department of Surgery, Scripps Mercy Hospital, San Diego, CA, USA

Jason Nam, MD Department of Medicine, Womack Army Medical Center, Fort Bragg, NC, USA

Michael Nurok, MD Department of Surgery, Smidt Heart Institute, Cedars-Sinai Medical Center, Los Angeles, CA, USA

Deven C. Patel, MD Division of General Surgery, Department of Surgery, Cedars-Sinai Medical Center, Los Angeles, CA, USA

Division of Thoracic Surgery, Department of Cardiothoracic Surgery, Stanford University, Stanford, CA, USA

Jason C. Pradarelli, MD Department of Surgery, Brigham and Women's Hospital, Boston, MA, USA

Edward Ray, MD Department of Surgery, Cedars-Sinai Medical Center, Los Angeles, CA, USA

Jordan E. Rogers, MS Department of Human Factors and Behavioral Neurobiology, Embry-Riddle Aeronautical University, Daytona Beach, FL, USA

Ali Salim, MD Harvard Medical School, Brigham and Woman's Hospital, Boston, MA, USA

Harry C. Sax, MD Department of Surgery, Cedars-Sinai Medical Center, Los Angeles, CA, USA

Randy Sherman, MD Department of Surgery, Cedars-Sinai Medical Center, Los Angeles, CA, USA

Daniel Shouhed, MD Department of Surgery, Cedars-Sinai Medical Center, Los Angeles, CA, USA

Bernadette McCrory, PhD Mechanical and Industrial Engineering, Montana State University, Bozeman, MT, USA

Dhivya R. Srinivasa, MD Department of Surgery, Cedars-Sinai Medical Center, Los Angeles, CA, USA

Benjamin W. Starnes, MD Department of Surgery, University of Washington School of Medicine, Seattle, WA, USA

Thor Sundt, MD Division of Cardiac Surgery, Corrigan Minehan Heart Center, Massachusetts General Hospital, Boston, MA, USA

Tsuyoshi Todo, MD Comprehensive Transplant Center, Department of Surgery, Cedars-Sinai Medical Center, Los Angeles, CA, USA

Mark Vrahas, MD Orthopaedics, Cedars-Sinai Medical Center, Los Angeles, CA, USA

Kristen L. W. Webster, PhD Department of Process Improvement, University of Louisville Health, Louisville, KY, USA

Karen N. Zaghiyan, MD Cedars-Sinai Medical Center, Los Angeles, CA, USA

Hanson Zhao, MD Department of Urology, Cedars-Sinai Medical Center, Los Angeles, CA, USA

Part I

Introduction

Introduction to Human Factors in Surgery

1

Bruce L. Gewertz

As surgeons in training, we became familiar with routine. The 10-minute scrub for our first case of the day, the ritual of draping, and the synchronized actions of surgeons, assistants, and scrub techs. The counting of sponges, needles, and instruments repeated twice. These rituals developed slowly over many years and were codified by all hospitals and slavishly examined by regulatory agencies. In the back of our minds, we knew they were introduced to lessen infections, improve the speed of operations, and avoid inadvertently leaving foreign objects inside operated patients. But, in truth, they were just part of our daily practice, like brushing our teeth. They were "hard wired" into our behaviors.

All that said, we knew that devotion to these practices was less than uniform. We all observed those who decided 10 minutes was just too long to scrub, and besides, they had other things on their mind. Sometimes a second count of the instruments was just too time consuming; after all, we looked into the wound and there was no way anything was left in there. And most of the time, nothing happened. The infection rates were low, hemostats did not appear in postoperative X-rays. And yet, every once in a while and in every hospital, bad things happened. A cluster of infections occurred in implanted heart valves, two patients developed abscesses from retained sponges, and the wrong finger was operated on.

These failures – and surely, they were failures of the worst kind – were not due to inherently faulty practices. They were, in the main, due to people not following those practices or guidelines. Possibly their behaviors also reflected larger, more systemic deficiencies including institutional demands that made surgeons rush through procedures, inefficient designs of the operating suites, or lack of training and supervision. But all resulted in people not following established protocols and putting patients at risk.

B. L. Gewertz (✉)
Cedars-Sinai Medical Center, Los Angeles, CA, USA
e-mail: Bruce.Gewertz@cshs.org

T. N. Cohen et al. (eds.), *Human Factors in Surgery*,
https://doi.org/10.1007/978-3-030-53127-0_1

The science of human factors is focused on investigating these disconnects and identifying solutions to remedy them. Human factors research began in other high-risk industries such as military operations, industrial sites, and aviation and has only been widely applied to medicine in the last 15 years. The field takes the most expansive view of the environment we work in and asks how that environment helps or hinders the behaviors of the people that work there. As research has evolved, much emphasis has been placed on more precisely quantitating these environmental factors and the attitudes and behaviors that contribute to safe behavior.

There are compelling reasons for incorporating more human factors analysis in our practices. For one, the pace of technology development in our fields has been accelerating. Whether surgeons are performing robotic surgery, endovascular procedures, or complex musculoskeletal instrumentation, the devices we use are intricate and constantly being upgraded. It is not uncommon to find manufacturers' representatives in our operating rooms every time the devices are deployed or implanted. Optimal interpersonal interactions between these nonphysicians and the operating surgeon are essential for safety and require heightened skill sets in communication, cooperation, and trust building.

Second, expectations for our work are ever increasing. Patients, families, and payors expect consistent and excellent outcomes even as we are performing complex surgery on older and sicker patients. Benchmarks for outcomes and readmissions as well as costs are widely available, and they drive all evaluations of our performances.

In this volume, we will examine how human factors principles can be applied to optimize care processes in surgery in general and in each major specialty. We hope to give readers a framework to analyze their own practices and improve the environment they work in. It is our sincere hope that implementing well-designed process improvements will deliver sustainable benefits to both patient health and physicians' well-being.

Part II

Human Factors

Human Factors Principles of Surgery

2

Tara N. Cohen, Eric J. Ley, and Bruce L. Gewertz

What Is Human Factors?

When working in a hospital, you may have heard the term "human factors" during a root cause analysis (RCA) meeting or from hospital leadership when discussing safety and efficiency. Without a formal definition, the concept often remains a mysterious lumping together of two words whose definitions are known separately, but not when joined. Human factors approaches have been utilized since the mid-1900s (some argue earlier); however, the field did not gain traction in healthcare until the publication of the well-known report, *To Err is Human*, by the Institute of Medicine [1]. Despite the recent proliferation of interest in human factors engineering among medical organizations, the majority of even the most well-meaning of individuals who reference the term usually have little idea of how a human factors approach is actually applied in healthcare.

Human factors (also referred to as ergonomics) has been formally defined as "the scientific discipline concerned with the understanding of interactions among humans and other elements of a system, and the profession that applies theories, principles, data and methods to design in order to optimize human well-being and system performance" [2]. Rather than focusing on individual challenges within an organization (e.g., redesigning a certain piece of technology) without plan or purpose, the goal of human factors is to analyze and improve the entire system by identifying and individually targeting its various components in a systematic way.

T. N. Cohen (✉) · E. J. Ley · B. L. Gewertz
Cedars-Sinai Medical Center, Los Angeles, CA, USA
e-mail: Tara.Cohen@cshs.org; Eric.Ley@cshs.org; Bruce.Gewertz@cshs.org

T. N. Cohen et al. (eds.), *Human Factors in Surgery*,
https://doi.org/10.1007/978-3-030-53127-0_2

A (Very) Brief History of Human Factors

A complete history of the field of human factors would require an entire book, so we will just provide a general and brief overview of the field's history. Interest in what we now call human factors arguably first arose as early as the fifth century BC, when the early Greeks used human factors principles to design tools, workplaces, and jobs. It was Hippocrates who first put down in writing the value of workplace design and tool arrangement during surgery. He was one of the first to argue that a surgeon's posture; the source of light in the room; instrument location; and surgical weight, size, and shape impact performance [3].

The late 1800s sparked the rise of *Taylorism*, or the scientific study of the worker, named after Frederick Winslow Taylor, a mechanical engineer interested in improving industrial efficiency. In one of his seminal studies of the Bethlehem Steel Company, Taylor realized that the efficiency of the entire organization could be improved if each man used a better shovel. Prior to Taylor's arrival, all of the tools in the factory fell under a "one-size-fits-all" model. Regardless of the task, be it breaking through dense, heavy substances or scooping light materials like ash, all workers used the exact same shovel. Taylor offered each worker eight specialized shovels that would be best designed for the task at hand. As a result of this change, worker daily output increased from 16 tons to 59 tons [4].

If you are familiar with the 1950 film "Cheaper by the Dozen," then you already know about this next group of scientists. The movie was based on the real-life story of Frank Gilbreth (one of Taylor's students) and his wife Lillian Gilbreth. The Gilbreths pioneered the modern incarnations of ergonomics and human factors (often experimenting on their own large brood of children), expanding upon Taylor's work to develop *time and motion studies* that aimed to improve efficiency by eliminating unnecessary motions. Their most well-known study involved reducing the number of steps and actions associated with bricklaying. Through this process, they reduced the number of motions it took to lay a single brick from 18 to 4.5, which boosted productivity from 120 to 350 bricks laid per hour. More relevant to surgery, the Gilbreths also applied their expertise to the operating room environment by analyzing video recordings of surgical procedures. They analyzed surgeons movements to identify opportunities to make work more efficient and less fatiguing. One of their major findings was that surgeons spent a great deal of time looking for their surgical instruments; as a result they recommended that instruments should be organized and presented in standardized and consistent patterns, a practice consistently applied today [5].

The terms "human factors" and "ergonomics" entered the contemporary lexicon during World War II. During this period, new and complex military machinery and weaponry were developed, placing higher cognitive demand on users. This was especially true in military aviation. Fully functional aircraft operated by the best-trained pilots were crashing to the ground. In fact, only one-third of US Army Air Corps pilot losses during this time were due to loss in combat, with the remainder occurring as a result of training crashes and operational accidents [6]. Researchers found that pilot error could be significantly reduced when cockpit design was taken into consideration and standardized controls were utilized. Over half a century later, researchers in the United Kingdom became some of the first to formally apply a human factors approach to surgery. Leval and colleagues [7] studied the relationship between surgical performance and outcomes in arterial switch operations and found that both major and minor events can lead to negative outcomes. Uncompensated major events (failures that were likely to have serious consequences for the safety of the patient (e.g., serious cannulation problems, failure to gain sufficient vascular access, ventilation errors)) were likely to lead to death, but could be avoided with appropriate human defense mechanisms. The more subtle and insidious minor events (failures that disrupted the surgical flow but did not have serious consequences for the patient in isolation (e.g., coordination problems, communication breakdowns, distractions)) were likely to go undetected and uncompensated by the team and their multiplicative effect was found to have a strong relationship with negative outcomes [7].

What Is a System?

Each of these early iterations of human factors has one thing in common: they highlight the importance of focusing on the system rather than individual performance. But what does it mean to focus on the entire system? How do we define a system? Human factors practitioners who work in healthcare often reference the Systems Engineering Initiative for Patient Safety (SEIPS) model when asked to describe what they mean by a system (Fig. 2.1) [8]. The SEIPS model was developed as part of the

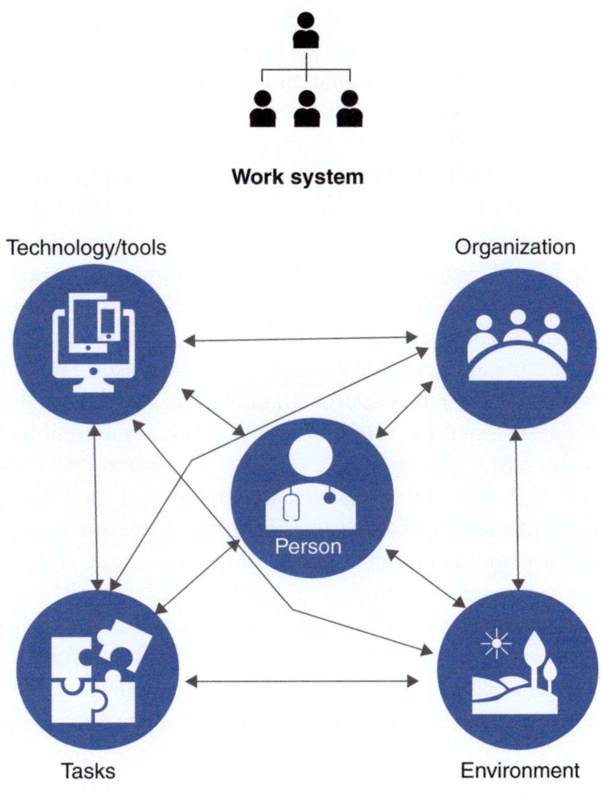

Fig. 2.1 The SEIPS model. (Adapted from Carayon et al. [8])

Systems Engineering Initiative for Patient Safety and was originally funded by the Agency for Healthcare Research and Quality (AHRQ). The SEIPS model maintains that healthcare professionals (e.g., surgeon, nurse, technician) work with other individuals to perform a range of tasks requiring the use of various tools and technologies, within given physical environments under specific organizational conditions. Factors impacting surgical performance can have several components: (1) the person – including teamwork/communication; (2) tasks; (3) tools/technologies; (4) physical environment; and (5) organizational conditions. None of these components are experienced in isolation – they are all part of an interacting and interlocking sociotechnical system in which the confluence of interactions produces various work processes which impact different outcomes related to satisfaction, safety, and quality. Notably, in 2013, the creators of SEIPS expanded and extended the model (SEIPS 2.0) to incorporate three concepts: configuration, engagement, and adaptation [9]. Additionally, among other clarifications, they differentiated between the internal environment (physical environment) and an external environment (societal, ecological, economic, and policy factors that occur outside of an organization). However, to keep things simple, we will use the original SEIPS model (shown in Fig. 2.1) when describing the role of human factors in surgery in this text.

What Does This Mean for Surgery?

While much progress has been made in reducing adverse events in healthcare, the overall rate of error remains high. A 2013 review of 14 studies analyzing surgical adverse events found that unintended injury or complication occurred in about 14.4% of all surgical patients and 5.2% of the total events were potentially preventable [10].

Errors made during an operation have been traditionally attributed to a surgeon's ability. By focusing on a surgeon's perceived skill, the number of contributing factors to conditions that allow for errors is marginalized. This narrow attribution disregards the many factors that are vital to maintaining safe and efficient performance in surgery and other high-risk industries. Oft-overlooked yet essential ingredients in building safe and efficient working environments include organizational culture, teamwork and communication, physical layout, interface design, usability, and cognitive abilities.

A human factors approach, unlike the conventional human-centered perspective, suggests that error is often the result of a combination of these various work system factors. Surgical teams are required to integrate progressively complex technology, communicate and coordinate among several multidisciplinary team members with differing levels of expertise, problem-solve on the spot to develop solutions for unforeseen patient challenges, and manage cost and time limitations that organizations demand. It is important to note that while most errors or adverse events occur when multiple factors break down the existing defense mechanisms in a system, there are rare occasions in which the human willfully disregards the rules and regulations and acts outside of the norm. These individuals are examples of exceptions to the norm which leadership should manage accordingly.

The Person

A human factors approach does not focus on the errors that a particular person makes; rather, human factors practitioners use expert and instinctual knowledge about human behavior, attitudes, and cognitions to understand and redesign systems and processes, so that errors are less likely happen in the future. The *person* part of the system focuses on the proactive identification of what fosters high-quality surgical performance, rather than highlighting surgical mistakes or developing reactive methods to address these missteps. The *person* component can involve any member of the surgical team (e.g., surgeon, nurses, anesthesiologists, technicians, and other staff). Perhaps most central to patient safety in surgery is an individual's ability to detect and recover from potential threats before they ever reach the patient, a skill described as *error management*. Historically, great surgeons were recognized based on their technical abilities, knowledge of the specialty, and diagnostic expertise. However, nontechnical abilities such as effective communication and individual leadership style also translate to safe, satisfied patients and better outcomes [11]. While some evidence suggests that certain leadership skills are innate, there are numerous ways to develop and improve upon these skills. For example, individuals can seek help from mentors, take part in institutional programs, attend leadership courses, or even obtain advanced degrees involving leadership and management.

Teamwork/Communication

Teamwork has been studied extensively in the context of surgery, with much of the research focused on specific disciplines and how to improve teamwork and performance in that unique discipline. Teams often interact with one another, or have smaller sub-teams, as well as larger overarching and overlapping teams. Teamwork-related factors can cause or prevent adverse events, and much research has gone into improving teamwork to prevent patient harm.

> Consider the following example from a case observation: during a cardiac surgery (involving a cardiac surgeon, an anesthesiologist, perfusionist and support staff), the surgeon commented: "I need you to go up" without explicitly referring to one person in the room. The perfusionist assumed the surgeon was talking to him and began to increase the flow of blood from the cardiopulmonary bypass machine to the patient. Simultaneously, the anesthesiologist believed the surgeon was talking to him and began to raise the head of the patient table. The surgeon, who was not expecting the head of the bed to rise during this point in the procedure, announced "whoa, what are you doing" to anesthesia. Luckily, this communication failure was caught before a catastrophic error occurred, but the situation could have been avoided entirely had the team communicated more effectively.

Common interventions that have alleviated communication failures include team training, checklist implementation, team briefings, and enacting stricter protocol-driven communication (e.g., standard formats like SBAR or IPASS). In one study, implementing a protocol-driven communication format decreased frequency of communication issues from 11.5 per case to 7.3 per case, on average

[12]. Interventions for communication failures in healthcare (e.g., team training and checklists) are also common for other teamwork competencies, and for teamwork and team performance in general. For example, simulation has been used to integrate training for both technical (e.g., dexterity) and nontechnical (e.g., leadership, communication, decision-making, error management, conflict management) skills.

Tasks

As operative procedures become more complex, surgeons are at a greater risk of work-related injury and even burnout (characterized by emotional exhaustion, depersonalization, and low personal accomplishment) [13]. Several studies have investigated the role of job demands in surgery on performance and safety, such as workload, time pressure, cognitive load, and attention, which have been grouped together into the category of "surgical task factors."

Physical workloads that can be described as excessive include prolonged muscular load, awkward and constrained postures, and/or repetitive movements, with task duration and strength requirements most impacting these factors in the goal of completing a task. In certain types of surgery, muscular fatigue from prolonged and awkward surgical postures has been seen to cause physical symptoms such as neck, back, and shoulder pain, as well as injuries in the hand and elbow. Cognitive load (or mental workload) refers to the proportion of attentional resources that a task or set of tasks demands. Tasks that are more difficult tend to be associated with higher workload, leaving little or no spare attention to respond appropriately to new or unexpected events, thereby increasing the likelihood of errors [14, 15].

Workload issues have been shown to relate to physician burnout, manifesting in increased medical errors, lower patient satisfaction, and decreased professional work effort. While there are several factors that contribute to physician burnout, high workload due to clerical tasks and documentation associated with the electronic health record (EHR) have become a major pain point [16]. For example, a time-motion study involving direct observation of over 50 physicians found that the average physician spent 49% of their time completing bookkeeping tasks. Even worse, physicians spent twice as long on EHR-related tasks than they did on clinical work [17]. Several solutions have been suggested to decrease harmful task-related factors in the surgical environment. With respect to physical and mental workload, recent literature has demonstrated the positive impact of intraoperative targeted stretching micro breaks (TSMBs) on surgeons' experienced pain and fatigue, physical functions, and mental focus [18, 19]. Perhaps more common, however, checklists to mitigate errors during stressful situations have seen a great deal of uptake. When well-designed and implemented under the correct circumstances, checklists can be incredibly useful. However, when designed or implemented inappropriately, checklists can cause additional issues such as "checklist fatigue."

Tools/Technologies

Participation in any surgical environment requires interaction with complex tools and advanced (or sometimes antiquated) technologies. Nowadays, tools and technologies used in surgery include the electronic medical record, medical devices, robots, automation techniques, virtual reality, and any other items you use in your daily activity to accomplish tasks. While tools and technology can improve surgical performance and patient care, they are often poorly designed and can cause harm by increasing errors or making work processes inefficient. Medical devices that are similar in design and purpose may not always function with the same user inputs. For example, laparoscopic surgery requires complex endostaplers to both divide bowel and create an anastomosis. Seemingly similar devices function very differently such that one device may require squeezing the handle firmly while another requires a handle double click. If the user is unfamiliar with the device requirements, then the bowel anastomosis may breakdown postoperatively. These miscues from devices can lead to catastrophic complications. Nearly half of all recalls of medical devices are due to design flaws, with certain devices being associated with dangerously high use error rates [20].

The introduction of new technology into the OR can lead to a range of intraoperative inefficiencies and risks. Prior to the implementation of new tools and technology, it is imperative that surgeons and other team members are prepared and trained on the potential hazards and new procedures associated with the tools. It is a necessity that training be included anytime a new tool or technology is implemented in the surgical system. Some have argued that stringent regulations, including audits of initial performance and comparison of standard approaches, should be required when new tools and technologies are introduced. A well-recognized approach to trialing these skills involves the use of medical simulation which can be used to investigate the effectiveness of new instruments with no impact to actual patients.

Physical Environment

Within the operating room (OR), the "environment" refers to the physical space, equipment, and individuals (staff and patients) in that space. While most OR team members have adapted to the ever-increasing complexity of the surgical theater, there are several factors beyond competency that have the potential to impact surgical performance and patient safety. Such contributing factors include lighting, temperature, noise, and physical layout of the room. Despite a vast increase in the number of instruments, equipment, and connecting wires better designed for efficient monitoring and treatment of surgical patients, the size and architectural layout of the OR typically remains unchanged. This has led to cluttered equipment and entangled lines and wiring (known as the *spaghetti syndrome*) [21]. When paired with the challenge of working with several multidisciplinary team members (including medical students, human factors researchers, and other visiting observers), a cluttered OR layout can restrict the movement of team members, hinder access and maintenance of lines and wires, and increase the risk of accidental line disconnection and other errors. Additionally, team member traffic in and out of the OR during surgery has been found to distract the operating surgeon [22].

Overcluttered environments hosting multiple team members and numerous pieces of equipment, each with its own alarm or alerting systems, can make for a noisy OR. Healthcare has more recently applied the "sterile cockpit rule" used in aviation to reduce nonessential activities and discussion during periods of high risk. When a structured sterile cockpit-driven protocol was introduced in cardiac surgery, there were significant reductions in communication breakdowns (e.g., inaccurate/incomplete information or the failure to share information or involve team members) [12].

Organizational Conditions

Most organizations have accepted the idea that whenever a human is involved with a process, error is inevitable. However, there are organizations operating in high-risk environments that continue to function at incredibly safe levels as compared with the average. These organizations are called "high reliability organizations" (HROs) and they design their work systems to anticipate risks and plan in advance for recovery from errors when they occur. HROs make a commitment to five values/actions: (1) *commitment to resilience* – the ability to be adaptable and bounce back from failure or upsets; (2) *sensitivity to operations* – paying of special attention to those on the front line who are doing the majority of the work; (3) *deference to expertise* – deferring to the experts (e.g., surgeons) rather than authority (e.g., administration); (4) *reluctance to simplify* – taking deliberate steps to create the most complete picture of a process or situation; (5) *preoccupation with failure* – treating any lapse or near miss as a sign that there might be something wrong with the system instead of just individuals [23].

An organization's culture has been found to play a substantial role in patient safety and even in surgical outcomes. In a cross-sectional study of 91 hospitals, those with a better safety climate overall had a lower incidence of patient safety indicators (indicators of potential patient safety events). Programs that support the union of hospital administrators, leaders, and front-line providers have been found to improve safety culture in healthcare organizations. Interventions such as TeamSTEPPS [24], Comprehensive Unit-based Safety Program (CUSP: a model for safety improvement focused on educating staff in the science of safety, identifying defects, engaging leaders, learning from defects, and implementing teamwork tools), [25] and executive walk rounds (frequent visits to patient care areas by individuals in leadership positions) [26] have been found to positively influence safety culture.

Human Factors Methods

This chapter serves as an introduction and overview of the assorted work system factors that should be considered when applying a human factors approach to surgery. Each of these factors and the methods used to study them, will be discussed in greater detail in the subsequent chapters. Due to the diversity of thought and scholarship within the field, numerous methods [27] have been applied in human factors approaches to improve safety and efficiency in healthcare [28]. With respect to surgery, data collection methods used to investigate each of the systems factors described above often include observations, interviews, and questionnaires.

Observational research approaches have been used to gather data about the current state of safety and performance in a complex system through the identification of intraoperative flow disruptions (deviations in the natural progression of a task that may compromise the safety of the task), the evaluation of task complexity, and the exploration of process steps [29]. Interviews (structured, semi-structured, and unstructured) can be used to gather information on several surgical topics such as usability, user perceptions, cognitive task analysis, errors, and opportunity for improvement. Focus groups allow us to gather similar information that can be collected from interviews but allows for group discussion that can be uniquely helpful in understanding group perceptions. Additionally, questionnaires have been implemented to investigate factors and attitudes that may influence surgical performance. Other methods such as cognitive task analysis, process charting, and accident analysis will be discussed in more detail throughout this text.

Conclusion

The involvement of a human factors approach is a requisite for future success at improving processes in an ever-changing surgical environment. The individual must be considered in conjunction with their team, environment, tasks, tools, and organization if safety, efficiency, and well-being are to be effectively studied and improved. By understanding how all the parts fit together as a whole, a human factors approach allows for a more comprehensive understanding of surgery.

Lessons Learned

- Human factors involves the application information about interactions between humans and various systems components to improve safety, efficiency, and well-being.
- The SEIPS model maintains that healthcare professionals (e.g., surgeon, nurse, technician) work with other individuals to perform a range of tasks requiring the use of various tools and technologies, within given physical environments under specific organizational conditions. Factors impacting surgical performance can have several components: (1) the person – including teamwork/communication; (2) tasks; (3) tools/technologies; (4) physical environment; and (5) organizational conditions.
- A human factors approach does not focus on the errors that a particular person makes; rather, human behavior, attitudes, and cognitions are uti-

lized to understand and redesign systems and processes, so that errors are less likely to happen in the future.

- Teamwork-related factors can contribute to or help to mitigate adverse events, and much research has gone into improving teamwork to prevent patient harm.
- When well-designed and implemented under the correct circumstances, checklists can be incredibly useful. However, when designed or implemented inappropriately, checklists can cause additional issues such as "checklist fatigue."
- Prior to the implementation of new tools and technology, it is imperative that surgeons and other team members are prepared and trained on the potential hazards and new procedures associated with the tools.
- When paired with the challenge of working with several multidisciplinary team members, a cluttered OR layout can restrict the movement of team members, hinder access and maintenance of lines and wires, and increase the risk of accidental line disconnection and other errors.
- High reliability organizations design work systems to anticipate risks and plan in advance for recovery from errors when they occur with a commitment to five values/actions: (1) *commitment to resilience*; (2) *sensitivity to operations*; (3) *deference to expertise*; (4) *reluctance to simplify*; (5) *preoccupation with failure*.
- Human factors data collection often includes observations, interviews, and questionnaires to investigate a system.

References

1. Kohn LT, Corrigan J, Donaldson MS. To err is human: building a safer health system. Washington, DC: National Academy Press; 2000.
2. International Ergonomics Association. What is ergonomics. IEA; 2020. Available from: https://www.iea.cc/whats/index.html.
3. Marmaras N, Poulakakis G, Papakostopoulos V. Ergonomic design in ancient Greece. Appl Ergon. 1999;30(4):361–8.
4. Meister D. The history of human factors and ergonomics. Boca Raton: CRC Press; 2018
5. Baumgar A, Neuhauser D. Frank and Lillian Gilbreth: scientific management in the operating room. Qual Saf Health Care. 2009;18(5):413–5.
6. Office of Statistical Control. Army Air Forces statistical digest (World War II). 1945:121.
7. de Leval MR, Carthey J, Wright DJ, Farewell VT, Reason JT. Human factors and cardiac surgery: A multicenter study. J Thorac Cardiovasc Surg. 2000;119(4):661–72.
8. Carayon P, Hundt AS, Karsh BT, Gurses AP, Alvarado CJ, Smith M, et al. Work system design for patient safety: the SEIPS model. BMJ Qual Saf. 2006;15(suppl 1):i50–i8.
9. Holden RJ, Carayon P, Gurses AP, Hoonakker P, Hundt AS, Ozok AA, et al. SEIPS 2.0: a human factors framework for studying and improving the work of healthcare professionals and patients. Ergonomics. 2013;56(11):1669–86.
10. Anderson O, Davis R, Hanna GB, Vincent CA. Surgical adverse events: a systematic review. Am J Surg. 2013;206(2):253–62.

11. Maykel JA. Leadership in surgery. Clin Colon Rectal Surg. 2013;26(4):254.
12. Wadhera RK, Parker SH, Burkhart HM, Greason KL, Neal JR, Levenick KM, et al. Is the "sterile cockpit" concept applicable to cardiovascular surgery critical intervals or critical events? The impact of protocol-driven communication during cardiopulmonary bypass. J Thorac Cardiovasc Surg. 2010;139(2):312–9.
13. Rotenstein LS, Torre M, Ramos MA, Rosales RC, Guille C, Sen S, et al. Prevalence of burnout among physicians: a systematic Review Prevalence of burnout among PhysiciansPrevalence of burnout among physicians. JAMA. 2018;320(11):1131–50.
14. Carswell CM, Clarke D, Seales WB. Assessing mental workload during laparoscopic surgery. Surg Innov. 2005;12(1):80–90.
15. Yurko YY, Scerbo MW, Prabhu AS, Acker CE, Stefanidis D. Higher mental workload is associated with poorer laparoscopic performance as measured by the NASA-TLX tool. Simul Healthc. 2010;5(5):267–71.
16. Shanafelt TD, Dyrbye LN, West CP. Addressing physician burnout: the way forward. JAMA. 2017;317(9):901–2.
17. Sinsky C, Colligan L, Li L, et al. Allocation of physician time in ambulatory practice: a time and motion study in 4 specialties. Ann Intern Med. 2016;165(11):753–60.
18. Park AE, Zahiri HR, Hallbeck MS, Augenstein V, Sutton E, Yu D, et al. Intraoperative "micro breaks" with targeted stretching enhance surgeon physical function and mental focus: a multicenter cohort study. Ann Surg. 2017;265(2):340–6.
19. Haynes AB, Weiser TG, Berry WR, Lipsitz SR, Breizat A-HS, Dellinger EP, et al. A surgical safety checklist to reduce morbidity and mortality in a global population. N Engl J Med. 2009;360(5):491–9.
20. Wiegmann DA, Eggman AA, ElBardissi AW, Parker SH, Sundt TM III. Improving cardiac surgical care: a work systems approach. Appl Ergon. 2010;41(5):701–12.
21. Brogmus G, Leone W, Butler L, Hernandez E. Best practices in OR suite layout and equipment choices to reduce slips, trips, and falls. AORN J. 2012;86(3):384–98.
22. Lynch RJ, Englesbe MJ, Sturm L, Bitar A, Budhiraj K, Kolla S, et al. Measurement of foot traffic in the operating room: implications for infection control. Am J Med Qual. 2008;24(1):45–52.
23. Weick KE, Sutcliffe KM. Managing the unexpected: sustained performance in a complex world. Hoboken: Wiley; 2015.
24. King HB, Battles J, Baker DP, Alonso A, Salas E, Webster J, Toomey L, Salisbury M. TeamSTEPPS™: Team strategies and tools to enhance performance and patient safety. In: Henriksen K, Battles JB, Keyes MA, et al., editors. Advances in patient safety: new directions and alternative approaches, vol. 3. Rockville: Agency for Healthcare Research and Quality; 2008.
25. Cooper M, Makary MA. A comprehensive unit-based safety program (CUSP) in surgery: improving quality through transparency. Surg Clin. 2012;92(1):51–63.
26. Frankel A, Grillo SP, Pittman M, et al. Revealing and resolving patient safety defects: the impact of leadership WalkRounds on frontline caregiver assessments of patient safety. Health Serv Res. 2008;43:2050–66.
27. Stanton NA, Salmon PM, Rafferty LA, Walker GH, Baber C, Jenkins DP. Human factors methods: a practical guide for engineering and design. 2nd ed. London: CRC Press; 2013. 656 p.
28. Carayon P, Wooldridge A, Hose B-Z, Salwei M, Benneyan J. Challenges and opportunities for improving patient safety through human factors and systems engineering. Health Aff. 2018;37(11):1862–9.
29. Catchpole K, Neyens DM, Abernathy J, Allison D, Joseph A, Reeves ST. Framework for direct observation of performance and safety in healthcare. BMJ Qual Saf. 2017;26(12):1015.

The Person: Individual- and Team-Level Factors Contributing to Safe and Successful Surgery

3

Jordan E. Rogers, Andrew C. Griggs, and Elizabeth H. Lazzara

Who is Involved in Surgery?

The act of surgery involves delivering surgical interventions to a patient to treat diseases, injuries, or improve other conditions. In order for surgery to be safely carried out, numerous highly specialized healthcare practitioners must work together to deliver care. As stated earlier in this book, "the person" component of the Systems Engineering Initiative for Patient Safety (SEIPS) model applies to any member of the surgical team: the surgeon, nurses, anesthesiologists, technicians, other staff, and even the patient.

Case Study

An 84-year male with obstructive jaundice and pancreatic cancer is a candidate for a Whipple procedure, which is a complex operation where the head of the pancreas and the first part of the small intestines are removed. This procedure typically takes between five and eight hours to perform. The surgical team on this patient's case consisted of a surgeon, resident, anesthesiologist, circulating registered nurse (RN), surgical technician, and a certified nursing assistant (CNA) who had not previously worked together within the same hospital, on the same type of operation.

During a delicate dissection along the posterior pancreatic head, the attending surgeon made a small incision in the superior mesenteric vein, a major blood vessel in the patient's abdomen, which caused a large bleed. The surgeon packed the area to stop the bleeding and then requested a hemoglobin test to determine if the patient might require a blood transfusion. However, the entire event was imperceptible to the

J. E. Rogers · A. C. Griggs · E. H. Lazzara (✉)
Department of Human Factors and Behavioral Neurobiology, Embry-Riddle Aeronautical University, Daytona Beach, FL, USA
e-mail: hilgersj@my.erau.edu; griggsa2@my.erau.edu; lazzarae@erau.edu

T. N. Cohen et al. (eds.), *Human Factors in Surgery*,
https://doi.org/10.1007/978-3-030-53127-0_3

remaining OR staff as the surgeon did not communicate that a bleed was occurring other than to request packing and lab work. The anesthesiologist drew blood from the patient's arterial line and gave the sample to the RN. The RN labeled the specimen and requested an order from the lab using the hospital's electronic medical record (EMR) software. The RN was not aware that all blood work sent during a major operation was considered STAT, so she requested it as routine in the EMR. The CNA who couriered the sample to the lab did not communicate the time-sensitive nature of the test to the lab personnel. Therefore, the lab received no indication that the order should be performed as quickly as possible. The surgeon was focused on repairing the hole in the superior mesenteric vein and completing the case. As the case progressed, the surgeon periodically asked for the results of the hemoglobin test and the RN would log into the EMR and state that it was not available. During the reconstruction of the pancreas to the small intestine, the patient's heart rate increased. The surgeon, rather than focusing completely on this important anastomosis, asked if the blood work was sent STAT, to which the nurse replied, "No, you did not ask for it STAT." The surgeon became frustrated because all labs should be sent STAT for her case; subsequently, she verbally belittled the RN and other team members. The RN called the lab, requested the order status, and was informed that the specimen had not been analyzed yet, which further frustrated the surgeon who then requested two units of blood without knowing the results of the lab work. Because the focus was now on missing blood work, the pancreas anastomosis leaked postoperatively, which led to significant morbidity and an extended hospital stay.

Overview

The nature of surgery has substantially evolved with the development of new medications, innovative techniques, and cutting-edge technology. For example, augmented reality, three-dimensional printing, genomic testing, nanotechnologies, and robotics are all changing the landscape of surgery. The introduction of novel techniques, equipment, and devices require changes in the surgical workforce; that is, individuals as well as teams must adapt and perform consistently and optimally.

To ensure that such innovations are implemented and mastered, attention must be directed toward the surgical team. Any deficits in individual and/or team performance can result in disastrous consequences for patients. To illustrate, recent research indicates that almost 60% of surgical adverse events are due to human error [1]. Consequently, modern surgical team members must be equipped with the requisite knowledge, skills, and attitudes, and surgical teams must be able to interact interdependently and expertly. Therefore, the purpose of this chapter is to synthesize what is currently known about individual- and team-level factors that lead to safe and successful surgeries. This chapter will define individual-level characteristics (i.e., orientation, well-being, skills, expertise, and familiarity) and team-level characteristics (i.e., collective efficacy, leadership, communication, and coordination) (Table 3.1), describe assessment methods, detail intervention efforts, and discuss relevance to the case study.

Table 3.1 Summary of discussed constructs and relevance to surgical teams

	Construct	Application to surgical teams
Individual-level constructs	*Orientation:* An individual's propensity to work with others	Individuals who are oriented toward teamwork may engage in beneficial team processes. Targeted team-building activities for surgical teams can promote orientation toward teamwork
	Well-Being: An individual's psychological, physical, and social health	Individual well-being (psychological, physical, and social) is linked with performance. Workplace redesign, team building, and improved safety practices can improve surgical team well-being
	Skills: An individual's technical or non-technical competencies	Surgical team members must exhibit both technical and non-technical skills in order to deliver effective care to patients. Surgical team members can improve their skills through training
	Knowledge and Expertise: An individual's areas of specialty	Knowledge and expertise facilitate individuals' decision making and strategies during surgery. Training interventions and repeated exposure to relevant taskwork may improve knowledge and expertise within surgical teams
	Familiarity with Team: An individual's level of familiarity with his or her team	Familiarity between surgical team members and with individuals outside of the surgical team can guide many cognitions that affect team performance, such as a shared awareness of individual team member capabilities
Team-level constructs	*Collective Efficacy:* A team's shared belief that they can accomplish their mission	Collective efficacy is related to greater team performance. High collective efficacy can be achieved in surgical teams when members positively perceive each other's intentions and competencies
	Leadership: The process of guiding team members toward the completion of their shared goals	Effective team leadership shapes team outcomes. Team training may help surgical team members to develop leadership skills and clearly define leadership roles and structure
	Communication: An exchange of information among individuals	Effective communication is needed to transform individual efforts into collective performance. There are a number of communication tools (e.g., checklists) that facilitate effective communication in surgical teams
	Coordination: The process of combining individual efforts into collective performance	High-performing teams are characterized by their ability to implicitly coordinate as a result of high task and team familiarity. This can be augmented in surgery through the use of *intact* teams

Methods for Measuring and Optimizing Individual- and Team-Level Constructs

To set the stage for our discussion of methods and approaches for studying and improving aspects of surgery related to "the person," several key components to situate the review must be presented. First, there are a plethora of individual- and team-level constructs that influence surgical performance and patient outcomes; however, the focus of the present review is on constructs that are malleable. For instance, one's personality can influence whether he or she is collectively oriented, but it is nearly impossible to alter one's personality. In order to maximize the utility of our review, we will focus on constructs that can be affected or improved through training or other interventions. Second, it is important to distinguish that there are different purposes behind the methods that will be discussed. There are methods that serve to *measure* constructs (e.g., skill assessment) and methods that seek to *affect* constructs through an intervention or change (e.g., team training).

Individual-Level Constructs

There are a variety of individual- and team-level factors that influence surgical team performance and patient outcomes. First, we will review constructs relevant to surgical teams at the individual-level, including orientation, well-being, skills, expertise, and team familiarity.

Orientation People value teamwork to different degrees; individuals can hold varying attitudes toward working with others and exhibit different levels of engagement with their team members. Theorists have characterized the attitude of wanting to work with others as *collective orientation* [2, p.52]. Collectivists are loyal to their team and exhibit preferences for team norms that facilitate group harmony [3]. Conversely, individuals who have individualistic attitudes exhibit greater orientation toward working alone. Such individual differences in orientation concerning teamwork can foster or preclude vital team processes and subsequently team performance. This is seen in the results of a meta-analysis performed by Bell (2007), which found significant effects for collectivism on team performance in studies across multiple field settings [3]. Attitudes concerning team orientation are typically assessed through subjective questionnaire methods and can be improved through targeted team-building interventions [4]. Concerning the above case study scenario, team orientation could have influenced each surgical team member's attitudes toward teamwork, such that members higher in collective orientation may have facilitated beneficial team processes such as conflict management or backup behavior.

Well-Being Individual well-being is another attitudinal factor that can influence team performance. In the abovementioned case study, the surgeon became increasingly distressed because a complication during the dissection was compounded with both a delayed blood test and a circulating nurse who was not familiar with how lab work is ordered. The postoperative pancreatic leak might initiate a subsequent review of why the complication occurred, which would contribute to additional distress and possibly even burnout.

Well-being refers to a holistic perspective of one's experience, functioning, condition, or state [5]. Well-being is a multidimensional construct. Grant, Christianson, and Price (2007) delineate three distinct forms: happiness (psychological well-being), health (physical well-being), and relationships (social well-being) [5]. Psychological well-being emphasizes the subjective experiences of individuals, such as the prevalence of positive or negative thoughts or perceptions of individual fulfilment. Physical well-being involves the intersection between work and physical health; it encompasses subjective experiences and objective measures of bodily health. Social well-being involves relational interactions and quality [5]. Well-being is linked to team performance, as individuals' psychological, physical, and social well-being can affect their ability and motivation to coordinate their efforts alongside their team. There are a variety of interventions that facilitate well-being in the workplace, such as workplace redesign, team-building exercises, and improving safety practices. However, organizations should be mindful of potential tradeoffs between dimensions of well-being as a result of an intervention, such as an increase in social well-being as a result of a team-building intervention accompanied by a decrease in psychological well-being due to reduced autonomy [5]. Physical well-being is typically assessed through various quantitative benchmarks of bodily health, while psychological and social well-being are frequently assessed through survey methods. In the case study above, the well-being of the surgeon and nurse was impacted by a difficult case, a lack of familiarity with how lab work was ordered, a lack of effective teamwork, and expressing frustrations inappropriately. Decreased well-being can lead to reduced trust, coordination, and cohesion among teammates.

Skills Compared to the contributions of a single individual, teams can leverage a greater variety of skills across multiple team members during task completion. As such, organizations often try to create teams of individuals with varying skills. Skills are often referred to as being technical or non-technical [6]. Technical skills refer to domain- or context-specific competencies necessitated by the current task or goal, while non-technical skills refer to interpersonal competencies that augment an individual's technical skills [6]. For example, a surgical team may need to rely on their clinical knowledge (technical skills) of a surgical procedure as well as effective communication strategies (non-technical skills) in order to successfully deliver care to a patient. Team training is an effective avenue for organizations to improve technical and non-technical skills [4], and there are a variety of methods that can be used to assess skills such as questionnaires or objective behavioral-anchor-based assessments. In the case study, deficits in technical skills could explain the accidental vessel laceration by the surgeon. Concerning non-technical skills, the delay in lab results is partially attributable to inadequate communication between team members and the nurse requesting blood work as routine rather than STAT.

Knowledge and Expertise Individual variance in technical and non-technical skills is also a reflection of differences in expertise. Experts are colloquially known as individuals with extensive knowledge or experience in a topic and, compared to novices, are characterized by differences in strategy and information management during task completion. Garrett, Caldwell, Harris, and Gonzalez (2009) delineated six dimensions of expertise concerning team performance: subject matter expertise, situational context expertise, interface tool expertise, expert identification expertise, communication expertise, and information flow path expertise [7]. Each dimension of expertise describes differences in cognition that take place during task completion. Expertise typically increases with time and exposure to relevant taskwork. Methods to assess expertise may include assessing an individual's declarative (i.e., simple recall of concepts, terminology) and/or procedural (i.e., recall of skill-based knowledge to inform decision-making) knowledge. Both declarative and procedural knowledge can be measured via written examination, while procedural knowledge specifically may be assessed by observing or proctoring the individual's behaviors. Team training is an effective intervention for the development of expertise because it provides increased exposure to taskwork in a risk-free environment (e.g., simulation-based training, and TeamSTEPPS) [4]. Expertise is highly related to surgical team performance and can influence the strategies and resources used during surgery. For example, expert surgeons may encounter less difficulty in determining which information or contextual factors they attend to most during surgery in comparison to a newly licensed surgeon. In the above case study, differences in expertise can assist in explaining the miscommunication surrounding the lab order. The surgeon assumed that her team would understand the order to be highly time-sensitive without explicitly stating that the request was a STAT order. Furthermore, the RN had the requisite technical skills to enter the request into the hospital's EMR appropriately but lacked the expertise to verify if the request should be STAT or routine.

Familiarity with Team Teams are not static entities and are composed of individuals who may or may not have previously worked together. One's familiarity with his or her team can contribute to emergent cognitive states by improving shared awareness of team member competencies and facilitating shared understanding of concepts (i.e., shared mental models) between team members [2]. These emergent cognitive states can have downstream effects on team performance by enabling greater utilization of available competencies within the team. Familiarity increases with time and reflects how team members perceive their knowledge of other team members' characteristics. As individuals begin their relationship with a team, they will exhibit greater preference for individuals whom they perceive as similar to themselves and for individuals with whom they are familiar [8]. As one's relationship with a team matures, he or she may exhibit preferences for those who he or she perceives as holding complimentary skillsets to him or herself and for team interactions that offer greater reward than cost [8]. Team familiarity can be assessed with surveys and improved through interventions such as team building, which provide opportunities to foster greater familiarity between team members [4]. Considering the case study, while the team has worked together for one year, a comparable level of familiarity did not exist between members of the surgical team and the lab personnel. Members of the surgical team did not have shared knowledge structures and awareness of individual competencies with the lab personnel, and, as a result, likely perceived them as dissimilar. Moreover, these deficits in familiarity and related cognitions place additional emphasis on effective communication as a mechanism to reduce the impact of a lack of shared understanding and awareness across the teams.

Team-Level Constructs

Hospitals and research organizations alike employ a number of approaches to evaluate and improve aspects of teamwork during surgery. The crux of these methods is to better understand and subsequently optimize how the work of teams is performed. This review of team-level factors will focus on collective efficacy, leadership, communication, and coordination, as these factors are influential and changeable.

Collective Efficacy Collective efficacy, the shared attitude or belief that the team encompasses the necessary resources and competencies to achieve their goals, is instrumental to safe and successful surgical care for a number of reasons. Similar to self-efficacy, collective efficacy drives the team's motivation, effort, and ultimately, performance. In the context of surgery, negative surgeon leadership behaviors (e.g., abusive supervision, or overcontrolling leadership) have been associated with lower ratings of collective efficacy [9]. Meta-analytic evidence points to a strong relationship between collective efficacy and team performance in teams with high interdependence [10]. This is especially noteworthy since surgical teams are characterized by a high level of interdependence. Collective efficacy is commonly measured through self-report methods in the form of interviews or questionnaires. Since past performance often begets future performance, collective efficacy is largely driven by a team's previous experiences together. Collective efficacy is mainly derived from an individual's perception of resources and team members' competencies and intentions; consequently, it may be improved through a number of avenues such as the effective provision of resources and team training. Considering this in light of the case study, had the team previously worked together, collective efficacy may have been improved by being aware of when the complication occurred, having a shared understanding that all labs are requested as STAT, and encouraging improved communication, while the surgeon's negative behaviors may have contributed to decreased collective efficacy.

Leadership Leadership, the way in which efforts are influenced and guided into performance, is vastly influential in surgical teams. In surgery, the surgeons are often considered to be the "de-facto" leaders due to their hierarchical status, extensive training, and expertise [11]. However, researchers have begun to study the phenomena of *shared leadership* in the context of surgery. Formative work illustrates that while surgeons conduct the bulk of leadership behaviors, other team roles are involved in influential leadership activities as well [12]. Regardless of the source(s), leadership is vital to guide team members toward the accomplishment of shared goals, as well as the development and maintenance of a safe interpersonal climate in which team members feel they are able to speak up and share concerns (i.e., psychological safety). Leadership can be assessed by tracking leadership behaviors as well as evaluating team members' perceptions. Fortunately, leadership can be taught and developed. Surgical teams may benefit from teamwork training that focuses on developing leadership skills (e.g., establishing goals, providing feedback, or solving problems) as well as clearly defining leadership roles for certain situations (i.e., if an anesthesia-related complication arises, then the anesthesia team member is the appropriate leader). With regard to the case study, the surgeon's frustration and belittlement of others characterizes ineffective leadership that likely contributed to decreased psychological safety.

Communication Many researchers posit that successful teams cannot function in the absence of effective communication; after all, communication is what drives key team functions such as situation awareness (i.e., maintaining an understanding of the current conditions and surroundings), mutual performance monitoring (i.e., team members overseeing each other's behaviors and work), and shared mental models. As such, the act of communication, both verbal and nonverbal, has been explored in highly complex work settings such as surgery. In order for individuals with differing backgrounds to combine their efforts, communication is needed. Tiferes, Bisantz, and Guru (2015) identified different techniques that are used to analyze communication in surgery, such as documenting the topic/theme (e.g., equipment, or patient), statement type (e.g., sharing information, or making a request), as well as breakdowns (e.g., message not accurate or not heard) related to communication [13]. Similar to other constructs discussed in this chapter, strategies and behaviors that support effective communication can be trained and learned. Fortunately, research on communication in surgery and other healthcare settings has resulted in actionable findings. For instance, checklists have been employed to promote standardized information exchange. Of note is the surgical safety checklist that is used perioperatively to ensure that relevant information (e.g., procedure type, location, known allergies) is communicated among the team. Researchers found that surgical teams who utilize structured communication tools such as the surgical safety checklist are less likely to experience negative outcomes such as patient complication and mortality rates [14]. Considering the case study, there were numerous instances of effective and ineffective communication. Notably, the surgeon failed to communicate the urgency of their lab tests. The RN, therefore, did not capture this in the lab request, and the CNA did not communicate this to the lab. If any of these individuals had more explicitly indicated the urgency level to the lab, the delay could have been avoided.

Coordination Coordination is integral to surgery as it is the process by which individual efforts are combined to yield collective performance. There are two primary types of coordination, *implicit* and *explicit*. Implicit coordination occurs when individuals anticipate each other's needs or next steps and work together seamlessly without reviewing or refreshing details such as specific responsibilities or timing related to the task. As evidenced in the above case study, the scrub tech knew exactly which instrument to hand to the surgeon during each step of the case without a specific request. Conversely, explicit coordination occurs when team members overtly explain or clarify aspects of their interdependency necessary for them to combine their efforts. When the surgeon had to review the steps to order blood work from the operating room, she lost focus during an important anastomosis. High-performing teams have been characterized by their ability to coordinate *implicitly* as this reflects high task and team familiarity. Researchers have touted the benefits of *intact* team scheduling for surgical teams to increase implicit coordination and overall functioning. *Intact* teams are characterized by consistent membership, compared to *non-intact* teams where membership varies. A surgeon's specific preferences may vary from physician to physician, so when team members are able to repeatedly work together, they gain familiarity with each other's needs and preferences. However, logistics such as scheduling and turnover present a major challenge to promoting *intact* surgical teams. In cases where intact teams cannot be formed, coordination can also be improved through team training as well as standardized practices. One strategy that teams can be trained on is *back-up behavior*, which is when team members "pitch in" to offer support to others when carrying out a task. Back-up behavior facilitates coordination, as it spans various roles and responsibilities and ultimately serves to ensure that all team tasks are completed. Considering the case study, coordination concerning the lab request was poor. The surgeon assumed that the RN and anesthesiologist were aware of the urgency as they processed the EMR and couriered the specimen. If the surgeon had overtly clarified the level of urgency, the delay may have been avoided.

Conclusion

With the average American undergoing 9.2 surgeries in their lifetime [15] and with a mounting number of clinicians entering the surgical workforce, individual- and team-level factors that lead to safe and successful surgical care are more important to consider now than ever before. Given the complexities associated with surgical care and the mandated multidisciplinary approach, consideration of these factors is both necessary and beneficial. This chapter reviewed several methods whereby researchers and practitioners alike can seek to better understand individual- and team-level constructs in surgery. In addition, this chapter outlined numerous strategies to bolster individual- and team-level competencies, such as the utility of individual and team training (both technical and non-technical), the usage of intact teams, leadership skill development and role clarification, and effective communication tools. The aim of this chapter is akin to the twofold objective of many of the methods discussed: to better understand and thereby improve surgical teamwork.

Lessons Learned/Personal Pearls

- Individual-level constructs such as orientation, well-being, skills, expertise, and team familiarity can impact performance and well-being.
- Team-level constructs including collective efficacy, leadership, communication, and coordination are influential and changeable.
- Team training has been found to improve various team-level constructs such as collective efficacy and communication.

References

1. Suliburk JW, Buck QM, Pirko CJ, et al. Analysis of human performance deficiencies associated with surgical adverse events. JAMA Netw Open. 2019;2(7):e198067. https://doi.org/10.1001/jamanetworkopen.2019.8067.
2. Salas E, Rosen MA, Burke SC, Goodwin GF. The wisdom of collectives in organizations: an update to the teamwork competencies. In: Salas E, Goodwin GF, Burke CS, editors. Team effectiveness in complex organizations: cross-disciplinary perspectives and approaches. New York: Taylor & Francis Group; 2008. p. 39–79.
3. Bell ST. Deep-level composition variables as predictors of team performance: a meta-analysis. J Appl Psychol. 2007;92(3):595–615. https://doi.org/10.1037/0021-9010.92.3.595.
4. Salas E, DiazGranados D, Weaver SJ, King H. Does team training work? Principles for health care. Acad Emerg Med. 2008;15(11):1002–9. https://doi.org/10.1111/j.1553-2712.2008.00254.x.
5. Grant AM, Christianson MK, Price RH. Happiness, health, or relationships? Managerial practices and employee well-being tradeoffs. Acad Manag Perspect. 2007;21(3):51–63.
6. Gordon M, Darbyshire D, Baker P. Non-technical skills training to enhance patient safety: a systematic review. Med Educ. 2012;46(11):1042–54. https://doi.org/10.1111/j.1365-2923.2012.04343.x.
7. Garrett SK, Caldwell BS, Harris EC, Gonzalez MC. Six dimensions of expertise: a more comprehensive definition of cognitive expertise for team coordination. Theor Issues Ergon Sci. 2009;10(2):93–105. https://doi.org/10.1080/14639220802059190.
8. Bell ST, Brown SG. Selecting and composing cohesive teams. In: Team cohesion: advances in psychological theory, methods and practice. Bingley: Emerald Group Publishing Limited; 2015. p. 181–209.
9. Barling J, Akers A, Beiko D. The impact of positive and negative intraoperative surgeons' leadership behaviors on surgical team performance. Am J Surg. 2018;215(1):14–8. https://doi.org/10.1016/j.amjsurg.2017.07.006.
10. Gully SM, Incalcaterra KA, Joshi A, Beaubien JM. A meta-analysis of team-efficacy, potency, and performance: interdependence and level of analysis as moderators of observed relationships. J Appl Psychol. 2002;87(5):819–32. https://doi.org/10.1037/0021-9010.87.5.819.
11. Stone JL, Aveling EL, Frean M, et al. Effective leadership of surgical teams: a mixed methods study of surgeon behaviors and functions. Ann Thorac Surg. 2017;104(2):530–7. https://doi.org/10.1016/j.athoracsur.2017.01.021.
12. Rydenfält C, Johansson G, Odenrick P, Åkerman K, Larsson PA. Distributed leadership in the operating room: a naturalistic observation study. Cogn Technol Work. 2015;17(3):451–60. https://doi.org/10.1007/s10111-014-0316-9.
13. Tiferes J, Bisantz AM, Guru KA. Team interaction during surgery: a systematic review of communication coding schemes. J Surg Res. 2015;195(2):422–32. https://doi.org/10.1016/j.jss.2015.02.034.
14. Haynes AB, Weiser TG, Berry WR, et al. A surgical safety checklist to reduce morbidity and mortality in a global population. N Engl J Med. 2009;360(5):491–9. https://doi.org/10.1056/nejmsa0810119.
15. Lee P, Regenbogen S, Gawande A. How many surgical procedures will Americans experience in an average lifetime? Evidence from three states. Massachusetts Chapter of the American College of Surgeons, 55th Annual Meeting. 2008. http://www.mcacs.org/abstracts/2008/p15.cgi. Accessed 31 Oct 2018.

Safe and Effective Use of Tools and Technology in the Operating Room

4

Tiffany Leverenz and Barbara S. Chaparro

Inroduction

The SEIPS model highlights tools and technology as one of the interacting components of the work system, which arguably is one of the only elements that involves usability engineering. Understanding the "user experience" of interacting with the tools and technology in the operating room is paramount to ensure safe and effective use, which directly affects patient outcomes. User experience can be defined as the overall experience a person has while interacting with a product or software application. For software, this may include the experience of using it on a variety of devices from a desktop computer to a tablet to a smartphone. For medical devices, the overall user experience may include usage under different procedures, for example, an operating table designed for a variety of procedures will have multiple positions for patient positioning based on the procedure type and the patient's risk factors. Proper user experience testing goes beyond the usability of a single tool or technology – it incorporates the tasks and the environment in which the tools may be used, understanding how users interact with them under different scenarios, and assesses potential errors that could influence patient safety.

T. Leverenz
Human Factors Engineer, Intuitive Surgical, Sunnyvale, CA, USA
e-mail: tiffany.leverenz@intusurg.com

B. S. Chaparro (✉)
Department of Human Factors and Behavioral Neurobiology, Embry-Riddle Aeronautical University, Daytona Beach, FL, USA
e-mail: Barbara.Chaparro@erau.edu

T. N. Cohen et al. (eds.), *Human Factors in Surgery*,
https://doi.org/10.1007/978-3-030-53127-0_4

Case Study

A 37-year-old male presented with a gunshot wound to the abdomen. Upon exploration, the surgeon determined that the missile went through the retrohepatic inferior vena cava, stomach, and spleen. In order to facilitate two teams working on either side of the table, a request was made for two bovies for electrocautery. Because the surgeon's instructions were not specific, rather than wheeling in a second bovie device into the crowded operating room, the circulating nurse plugged a second bovie into the initial unit. Unfortunately, and unbeknownst to the newly hired circulating nurse, two bovies cannot be connected to one device and used simultaneously. At the beginning of the case, only one bovie was used at a time and no disruptions in the case occurred. However, when simultaneous electrocautery was attempted, neither bovie worked. The surgeon asked the team to troubleshoot why the bovies were not working. Maybe it was the grounding pad? The circulating nurse confirmed the grounding pad was attached appropriately. As one bovie was then used successfully, no problem was identified. The liver mobilization progressed for a few minutes until both bovies were again used simultaneously. The case was stopped while there was significant bleeding. The patient was packed, and it was subsequently noted that only one bovie generator was in the room so a second one was obtained and the case progressed.

The operating room is a busy and demanding environment for everyone involved in a procedure. Clinical workers need to understand their own job and the tools and technology they interact with but also their team members' responsibilities. A typical operating room is filled with equipment, such as the surgical and back tables, lights, booms, and multiple monitors. It is also filled with people who make up the surgical team, typically including the surgeon, an anesthesiologist, a first assist, a circulating nurse, a surgical tech, and potentially others depending on the case. At times, simple instructions can be unclear with devasting results. The procedure dictates the amount of equipment needed, which may include many medical devices, imaging equipment, or even a robotic surgical system. These tools and technology often need to be physically moved and set up by the surgical staff prior to a case for optimal placement to build the sterile field.

Figure 4.1 illustrates a typical operating room setup with tools and technology labeled by number as well as the positions in which members of the team might be located.

Let us consider the circulating nurse's typical experience as an example of how tools and technology factor into the efficacy of their role. Before a case, the circulating nurse obtains and tracks supplies and sets up the operating room. They need to help the surgical (scrub) tech open surgical packages or kits, help the sterile staff with their gowns, and prep the patient. Throughout the procedure, they collaborate with the surgical team and coordinate with other departments as necessary, completing non-sterile tasks, such as documentation in the electronic medical record (EMR) system and interacting with medical devices, and toward the end of the procedure, coordinate for the current patient to be taken to recovery and prepare the next patient for surgery. If anything goes wrong with a device during a procedure, the circulating nurse is typically the one to troubleshoot since they are non-sterile. If the surgeon's

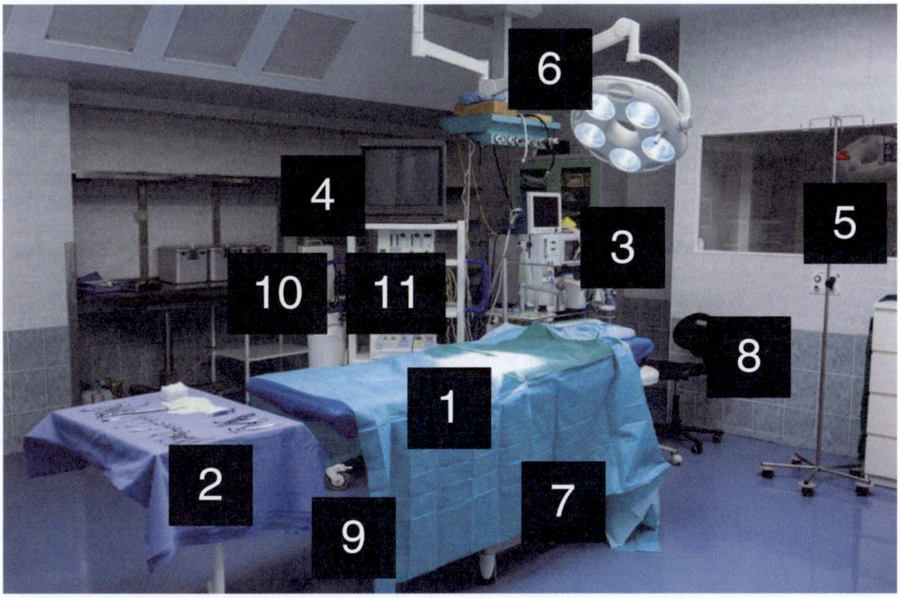

Fig. 4.1 Typical OR setup. Positions 1 through 11 are as follows: (1) surgical table; (2) additional table with surgical instruments and supplies; (3) anesthesia cart; (4) laparoscopy tower, which typically has a monitor, video and light monitors/equipment, an insufflation unit, and possibly an electrosurgical generator; (5) IV stand; (6) surgical light; (7) surgeon; (8) anesthesiologist; (9) surgical technician; (10) circulating nurse; (11) first assist (Designed by peoplecreations/Freepik)

pager goes off, the circulating nurse must answer for them. At each step from pre-op to post-op, the circulating nurse interacts with 25 or more different tools and technology in many different ways – from opening packaging to assembling a device with medication, to using the device per instructions, then documenting everything in the EMR. This routine is typical for even the most mundane surgery. Many surgeries, however, do not always go as planned. New surgical kits are sometimes needed, or new equipment needs to be set up mid-surgery. This adds a new level of complexity and responsibility to the team operations.

New tools and technologies are constantly being developed to enhance surgical teams, their tasks, and their performance. However, it is a common misconception that new technology offers a guaranteed advantage. How can we assess if a new tool or technology will make operations more efficient, or if it is safe for use? How do we know whether the investment is worth it? This is where human factors professionals can help.

Methods

There are many ways to assess the tools and technology for use in the operating room with varying degrees of complexity. Human factors professionals use techniques like workflow analysis, ethnography, heuristic evaluation, and

Table 4.1 Common human factors methods in medicine

Method	Description	When to use
Workflow analysis	Structured analysis of users in an environment with the focus on how they complete the tasks necessary for their job, how they interact with others, how they navigate their environment, and how they interact with technology	Early to understand typical workflow patterns of a single or group of users; understand interactions, use of technology, and tools to complete a task or set of tasks
Ethnography	Observational analysis of users in their natural setting/environment	Early to learn about the many roles and complexities of the operating room environment
Heuristic evaluation	Expert review of design to identify usability issues that can be fixed early	Early and often throughout the design process. Can be used to identify issues that can be fixed prior to testing users
Usability testing	Testing the learnability, ease of use, and satisfaction with representative end users	Throughout the design process to detect and correct problems based on user interaction with the system, device, or process

usability testing to assess the efficacy of tools and technology as well as to inform their design and redesign. The method employed depends on the research question at hand (Table 4.1). Workflow and ethnographic methods may be used as exploratory methods to better understand a certain role in the operating room, while heuristic evaluation and usability testing may be used to evaluate a particular tool or system both from an expert's and an end user's perspective.

Workflow Analysis

Thinking again about the circulating nurse's role in the operating room, we are reminded of the complexity of the tasks and necessity to think quickly under stressful situations. Workflow analysis is a technique that allows us to analyze different users with the focus on how they complete the tasks necessary for their job, how they interact with others, how they navigate their environment, and how they interact with technology. No new technology should be introduced to the operating room environment without this detailed understanding.

For example, suppose a surgeon enters the operating room and asks for additional equipment that was not originally anticipated by the circulating nurse. The circulating nurse becomes overwhelmed, as he is asked to obtain additional supplies while managing his very busy workload. Simultaneously, the surgeon becomes frustrated as she is waiting for the supplies and is unsure why there is a hold up. In an effort to mitigate these issues, the OR staff is interested in using a new electronic checklist that can be edited by surgeons the day prior to surgery and helps to ensure that all necessary equipment is pulled for the case. While this electronic checklist may appear to be helpful in isolation, its impact must be

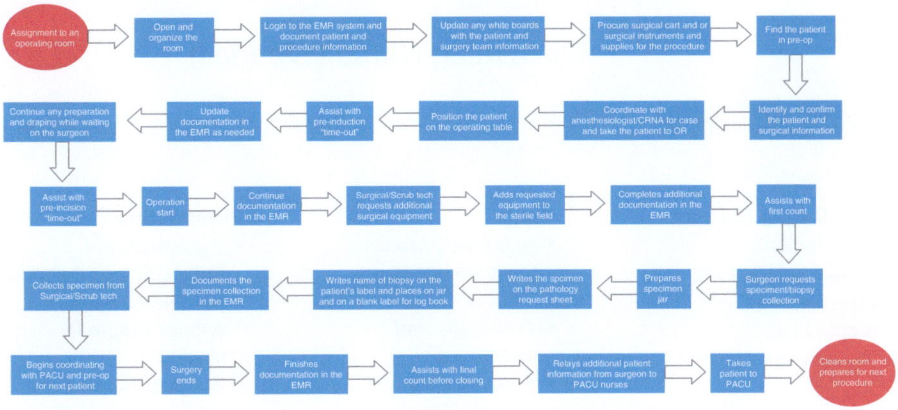

Fig. 4.2 Sample workflow for circulating nurse from pre- to post-op

considered in the context that it will be used, namely the operating room during various surgeries. Workflow analysis can be done to determine where, in the typical task flow, a new technology could be introduced. Figure 4.2 shows a sample workflow for a circulating nurse from pre- to post-op. Seeing a context in which a new tool may be introduced helps to understand how it may fit, or not fit, into the flow with other tools and technologies.

Ethnography Analysis

Ethnographic research has been growing in the healthcare field and a unique application of this is through design ethnography. This extension of the traditional anthropology method consists of similar methods, such as observation and interviews, to better understand end users' needs and preferences while also documenting keys aspects of their environment [1]. The goal of this analysis concerning tools and technology is to capture a "day-in-the-life" of a user and an appreciation of what works well and not so well. Additional stakeholders can be included in this process as well, for example, the entire surgical team that works with the circulating nurse discussed earlier. One outcome of this analysis is a representation of the "typical" user in each role as a persona (Fig. 4.3). A persona includes the typical characteristics of the typical user in that role, their tasks and responsibilities, their goals, and frustrations. Knowing this information helps the human factors researcher understand where improvements can be made to streamline processes and increase efficiency and overall satisfaction for each role.

Heuristic Evaluation Heuristic evaluation is a method that can be used to assess a device, system, or software based on a set of principles. Three to five expert evaluators use the heuristics as a guide throughout assessment. The original heuristic set developed by Nielsen and Molich [2] consisted of nine categories, with a tenth category

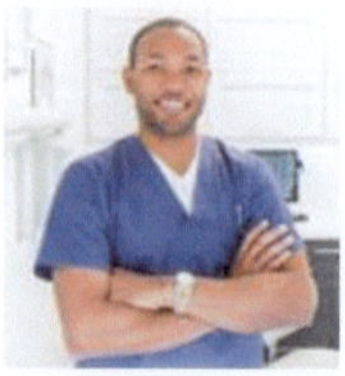

Circulating Nurse (Wendell)

Tasks During Surgery
- Prep Patient
- Gather surgical kits
- Help scrub tech; prepare kits
- Ready tools/EMR
- Assist team with non-sterile tasks

Goals
- Accurately predict tool/tech needs for surgery
- Anticipate staff needs
- Keep surgery running smoothly
- Be ready for the unexpected

Frustrations
- Equipment not responding as it should
- Kit doesn't have enough suture for closing
- Surgical kits needed not readily available
- Communication with surgeon is poor

Fig. 4.3 Sample persona of a circulating nurse's typical tasks, goals, and frustrations during surgery (Designed using resources from Freepik.com)

added later [3] (Table 4.2) and is still one of the most popular sets used today. Over the years, researchers and practitioners have adapted Nielsen's heuristics for other domains, including medical devices [4]. Additionally, heuristic checklists consisting of yes/no questions pertaining to design elements have been developed to increase clarity and obtain reliable results within this method. These checklists have been developed for mobile devices [5], accessibility [6], and clinical decision support mobile applications [7]. Although adapted for mobile devices, many of the questions in the decision support checklist [7] apply more generally to clinical decision support tools and technology that could be used in the operating room. Table 4.3 depicts a sample of such questions along with their heuristics and outcome category. Note that a new Clinical Decision Support category was added to Nielsen's for medical decision support applications [7]. The value of the checklist is that it allows evaluators to simply sum the "Yes" and "No" violations to assess the strengths and weaknesses of the technology.

Using a checklist like this early in the design of the tool/technology or evaluation process can facilitate the decision whether the tool or technology will actually be useful in the operating room context. Will it actually minimize errors and decrease the workload of the medical team user? Note that the heuristic evaluation is conducted by experts in human factors and/or the surgery domain and is therefore speculative. While this technique has been shown to be very helpful and predictive of usefulness, heuristic evaluations are not a replacement for traditional usability testing which involves actual users of the tool/technology. We all know that human behavior is not always predictable!

Usability Testing Perhaps the most popular approach to ensure ease of use and safety of tools and technology is usability testing. This is a procedure whereby representative users are brought into a controlled, yet representative, environment to test

Table 4.2 Usability principles or heuristics proposed by Nielsen (1995)

Heuristic	Description
Visibility of system status	The system should always keep users informed about what is going on, through appropriate feedback within reasonable time
Match between system and the real world	The system should speak the users' language, with words, phrases, and concepts familiar to the user, rather than system-oriented terms. Follow real-world conventions, making information appear in a natural and logical order
User control and freedom	Users often choose system functions by mistake and will need a clearly marked "emergency exit" to leave the unwanted state without having to go through an extended dialogue. Support undo and redo
Consistency and standards	Users should not have to wonder whether different words, situations, or actions mean the same thing. Follow platform conventions
Error prevention	Even better than good error messages is a careful design which prevents a problem from occurring in the first place. Either eliminate error-prone conditions or check for them and present users with a confirmation option before they commit to the action
Recognition rather than recall	Minimize the user's memory load by making objects, actions, and options visible. The user should not have to remember information from one part of the dialogue to another. Instructions for use of the system should be visible or easily retrievable whenever appropriate
Flexibility and efficiency of use	Accelerators – unseen by the novice user – may often speed up the interaction for the expert user, such that the system can cater to both inexperienced and experienced users. Allow users to tailor frequent actions
Aesthetic and minimalist design	Dialogues should not contain information which is irrelevant or rarely needed. Every extra unit of information in a dialogue competes with the relevant units of information and diminishes their relative visibility
Help users recognize, diagnose, and recover from errors	Error messages should be expressed in plain language (no codes), precisely indicate the problem, and constructively suggest a solution
Help and documentation	Even though it is better if the system can be used without documentation, it may be necessary to provide help and documentation. Any such information should be easy to search, focus on the user's task, list concrete steps to be carried out, and not be too large

Table 4.3 Sample heuristic checklist items for a medical decision support tool

Checklist question	Heuristic	Outcome category
Are processes/tasks simplified as much as possible without compromising the process in any way?	Recognition rather than recall	Memory load reduction
Is content updated regularly to the most recent clinical guidelines?	Clinical decision support	Patient safety
Does the application provide essential alerts when necessary? (e.g., drug interaction alert if two separate drugs with allergies are entered, alert of age if inappropriate drug dosing is chosen and age is known, etc.)	Clinical decision support	Clinical workflow

specific elements of a design and provide subjective feedback. The test is structured based on a set of usability goals. For example, suppose a hospital is assessing the efficacy of a new time-out checklist in the operating room. This tool will be a replacement to an existing checklist that has been reported to be cumbersome to use. The usability test is structured to compare user performance and satisfaction between the two tools. Researchers track performance objectively through metrics such as time on task, number of steps, and success rate for each tool. Subjectively, participants provide comments on their experience using the tools. This objective and subjective data is then combined to provide a relative comparison of the tool effectiveness.

Almost 20 years ago, the Federal Drug Administration (FDA) began providing guidance for quality manufacturing process and quality system regulation for all medical devices and now requires usability testing as part of the premarket submission for 510k clearance [8]. Their guidance document is meant to help industry manufacturers design safe, effective products by minimizing use errors resulting in harm. This type of usability testing is preceded by a usability risk analysis that identifies potential hazardous situations that are then mitigated within the design. These mitigations are then tested during human factors usability formative testing for their effectiveness, and any new risks identified are added to the analysis, addressed in the design, and tested in the next round of formative testing. Summative usability testing is conducted with the final design and the results are submitted as part of a larger report and submission to the FDA.

The abovementioned methods are conducted outside the operating room environment as controlled studies, but it is equally important to conduct field studies within the operating room. Case observations and time motion studies can be used to evaluate workflow, communication, interruptions, and teamwork to identify how tools and technology use can be optimized to increase safety and efficiency for pre-, intra-, and postoperative processes.

Future Technologies and Considerations

Just understanding the complexity of the role of the circulating nurse, surgeon, and other team staff in a typical surgery leads to the question on how technology could be used more to make this process and workflow even more efficient. New technologies including voice recognition and head-mounted mixed reality have been proposed for the operating room setting (Fig. 4.4). Given the sterile environment, use of hands-free methods of communication, enhanced imagery, data look-up, and data entry appear to be promising. They also introduce the potential for new problems and inefficiencies, however. Imagine the following scenarios and potential pros and cons:

- A surgeon uses mixed reality glasses during surgery that displays patient data or pager call information upon voice request.
  - Pro: surgeon no longer requires circulating nurse to complete the task, so this task is completed more efficiently.

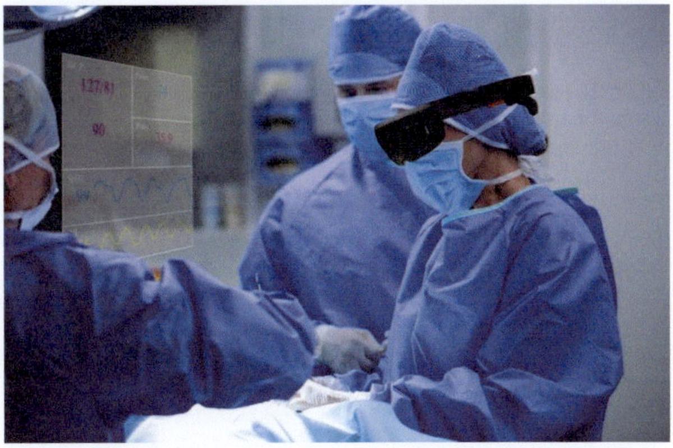

Fig. 4.4 Mixed reality glasses provide virtual patient information during surgery (Designed by peoplecreations/Freepik)

  - Con: the augmented patient data and/or pager information is superimposed on top of the patient body, obscuring the surgical field, dividing surgeon's attention and focus.
- A surgeon uses voice recognition software to display patient data on a computer monitor during surgery.
  - Pro: patient data is displayed upon command in an accurate and easy to view display, which aids the surgeon in decision-making.
  - Con: voice recognition software is not 100% accurate and results in repeat commands, error potential, and increased frustration in addition to divided attention to the surgery task being conducted.

Application of human factors methods and empirical research is needed to fully understand the likely outcomes of these scenarios in the operating room environment. Maintaining a focus on the end users of the tools and technology, whether it be through observation on the job or empirical testing in a simulation environment, is paramount to successful implementation.

Lessons Learned/Personal Pearls

- It is critical to understand the workflow and surgery environment before new tools or technology are introduced in the operating room.
- Ethnographic methods (observation, interviews) can be used to understand the interaction of the human operators and the technology.
- Expert evaluation of a new tool or technology can be done quickly by human factors and/or surgery specialists.
- Usability testing with representative users in a simulated environment should be conducted to truly understand the effect of the technology on user effectiveness, efficiency, and satisfaction.
- Futuristic technologies, such as mixed reality, may provide efficiency enhancements in some situations but must be assessed carefully to understand if they introduce new problems.

References

1. Mohedas I, Sabet Sarvestani A, Daly SR, Sienko KH. Applying design ethnography to product evaluation: a case example of a medical device in a low-resource setting. Proceedings of the 20th International Conference on Engineering Design (ICED15), Milan, Italy, 2015.
2. Nielsen J, Molich R. Heuristic evaluation of user interfaces. Proceedings of the SIGCHI conference on Human factors in computing systems Empowering people – CHI '90. 1990.
3. Nielsen J. 10 usability heuristics for user interface design 1995. Available from https://www.nngroup.com/articles/ten-usability-heuristics/.
4. Zhang J, Johnson TR, Patel VL, Paige DL, Kubose T. Using usability heuristics to evaluate patient safety of medical devices. J Biomed Inform. 2003;36(1–2):23–30.
5. Yáñez Gómez R, Cascado Caballero D, Sevillano JL. Heuristic evaluation on mobile interfaces: a new checklist. Sci World J. 2014;2014:19.
6. Mi N, Cavuoto LA, Benson K, Smith-Jackson T, Nussbaum MA. A heuristic checklist for an accessible smartphone interface design. Univ Access Inf Soc. 2014;13(4):351–65.
7. Leverenz T. The development and validation of a heuristic checklist for clinical decision support mobile applications. Doctoral dissertation, Wichita State University, 2019.
8. Applying human factors and usability engineering to medical devices. Guidance for industry and Food and Drug Administration staff. Document issued on February 3, 2016. Available from, https://www.fda.gov/media/80481/download.

Work System Tasks: Blending Art and Science

5

Bethany Lowndes and Bernadette McCrory

The Task

In the work system, the tasks performed by the surgeon and surgical team require a blend of art and science. Whether the procedure is a routine and high-volume procedure or a nonroutine and novel procedure, surgeons must navigate various anatomical and pathological differences that demand a high level of technical skill, cognitive and physical capacity, applied clinical knowledge, and ingenuity. Unlike many industrial fields including manufacturing and aviation, from which human factors principles and methods evolved, task standardization cannot supersede the necessary autonomy and adaptability required to accommodate patient variability and achieve optimal outcomes for patient care, safety, and satisfaction. However, integrating standard procedures can improve elements of patient safety as organizations strive for efficiency to balance resources and meet business goals [1]. Yet, standard procedures must not induce an unsustainable workload for the users. If the physical and cognitive demands (or workload) of the task exceed the capacity of the surgical team, surgical safety and efficacy will suffer. It is through task analysis and work design—as a part of the surgical process—that this balance between standardization and flexibility can be best established and workload can be managed.

This chapter (1) provides an example of how the task influences workload, performance, and outcomes as a part of the work system; (2) demonstrates how human factors professionals define and study surgical tasks; and (3) describes research methods used to break down and measure the task.

B. Lowndes (✉)
Department of Neurological Sciences, University of Nebraska Medical Center, Omaha, NE, USA
e-mail: Bethany.lowndes@unmc.edu

B. McCrory
Mechanical and Industrial Engineering, Montana State University, Bozeman, MT, USA
e-mail: bernadette.mccrory@montana.edu

T. N. Cohen et al. (eds.), *Human Factors in Surgery*,
https://doi.org/10.1007/978-3-030-53127-0_5

Example of Task-Specific Surgical Workload

Cholecystectomy is a common and generally routine procedure performed at hospitals of varying levels and capacities from community hospitals to quaternary care hospitals. Decades ago, the technique advanced from an open to a laparoscopic technique, allowing patients to benefit from reduced bleeding and pain, improved recovery time, and improved cosmesis [2]. To achieve these patient benefits associated with minimally invasive surgery (MIS), the work system needed to support the new processes associated with the MIS technique. Transition from open to laparoscopic cholecystectomy (LC) involved many of the tasks within the procedure process. The MIS technique also had overall implications for the work system.

For the transition to LC, several changes occurred within the surgical work system. Fundamentally, LC separated the surgical team members distally from the operative field, resulting in no tactile/physical contact with tissues, which required novel instruments to recreate the "feel" of open surgery in LC. This new, diverse instrumentation must be surgeon-selected by case or procedure type, sterilized, and prepared prior to the procedure, altering the preoperative phase of the surgical process. The physical environment and instrumentation transitioned to accommodate all team members working in tight proximity, manipulating advanced instrumentation and requiring visualization of the intra-abdominal operative field via the laparoscopic camera. The role-based responsibilities on the surgical team adjusted requiring less tissue retraction, but now necessitated laparoscopic camera operation for the duration of the procedure. Many of the steps including placement of the trocars (ports for the laparoscopic tools), insufflation of the abdomen for surgical working space, and dissection/removal of the gallbladder all differ from an open technique. Surgical trainees also had to be trained on the new technique. Over about two decades, the tasks associated with LC became routine with training, technology, and the surgical environment. Despite the increase in some workload measures for the surgeon and surgical team [3, 4], the work system evolved to meet the needs of the patients.

To continue improving care for the patients, laparoendoscopic single site (LESS) surgery—an advanced MIS technique—demonstrated promise of improved patient outcomes. Most notably, patient cosmesis was potentially improved by using only a single incision in the umbilicus compared to the multi-incision laparoscopic technique. While the literature on patient outcomes associated with LESS were limited, workload between the two techniques remained broadly undiscussed.

A randomized control trial (RCT) comparing LESS to LC [5] followed 48 (23 LESS) cases for an assessment of patient outcomes associated with each technique. In collaboration with the surgical team, researchers studied the workload for these two techniques and determined that workload during LESS exceeded the appropriate capacity to be sustainable without negative complications for members of the surgical team [6, 7]. The surgeons experienced higher physical and cognitive workload, especially around the critical phase of bile duct clipping [6]. While there was a similar workload experienced across some members of the team, including the surgical assistant and resident, the surgical technician and circulating nurse did not report a similarly high cognitive or physical workload [5]. It was expected that the workload would vary by role; however, a substantially lower workload may lead to task disengagement by surgical team members and prevent the team cohesion required to meet shared goals [4]. Additionally, with the workload above a threshold that is sustainable for long procedures or multiple cases in a day, surgeons, surgical assistants, and residents are at risk of injury, experiencing an error, or work burnout [3].

The results of the RCT did not support LESS as a superior alternative to LC with LESS resulting in no significant difference in bleeding and an increase in post-operative pain [5]. With a higher workload and failing to achieve the desired patient outcomes, the surgical team decided not to continue performing manual LESS procedures; instead, they opted to complete LC or robotic LESS procedures moving forward.

Surgical Tasks

A surgical *task* is an action carried out by the people within the work system as part of the surgical process. With advanced techniques and technologies, the tasks within surgery have become more numerous and further divided among more team members. Due to specialization of team role and procedure types within surgery, the tasks are often more repetitive and demanding on the surgeon and team members. There are many examples of task-related injuries [3] and errors [8] associated with surgery and resulting in negative consequences for patients and surgical team members. Human factors researchers focus on fitting the task and overall work system to the person in order to avoid these errors and reduce the risk of injury.

Surgical Task Factors and Task Implications

As mentioned in Chap. 2, the surgical task factors include task difficulty, complexity, variety, and ambiguity. Each factor describes an element of variability between and within different surgical procedures. A breast biopsy is not as complex as a bilateral mastectomy. During a bilateral mastectomy, the dissection of the more involved breast will have a higher difficulty level compared to the less involved breast. Between two different bilateral mastectomy procedures, one case could be more difficult due to patient anatomy or the size of a mass. Patients with a high BMI can change the orientation of the surgical team standing around the patient to access the surgical site, and the physical requirements for tissue retraction during open procedures can be much higher. These differences from case to case have a direct impact on the surgical tasks and the workload for the surgeon and surgical team.

The surgeon and surgical team must have the capacity to meet the demands of the task. When the workload is too high, the demand cannot be met and errors or injuries can occur. During the study and design of tasks, workload is the main consideration to fit the job to the human user. These physical and cognitive demands placed on the user are influenced by the other elements of the system. A well-designed surgical grasper can have a lower grip strength requirement and therefore reduce physical workload. Optimal visualization of the surgical site paired with ideal triangulation of instrumentation can reduce cognitive burden for surgeons. When workload remains at a sustainable level, the users are less likely to experience errors and have spare capacity to handle unexpected events.

Human Factors Approach to the Task

Within the field of human factors, the task is studied as a more basic element of the process in order to measure system function and interactions. When studying the task—or actions—within a work system, it is easy to include aspects of *what* occurs and *when* the steps take place. Surgical policies and procedures often define what should occur during the tasks and timing. Both are often dependent upon clinical resources and operational constraints. During a task analysis, the task can be further studied as a part of the system to analyze *what* resources are required for the task, *how* and *why* steps take place, and *who* completes the steps. As introduced in Chap. 2, the human factors approach studies the work system with the human at the center of the system. These "humans" carrying out tasks must have the capacity for completion. It is important to consider *who* is completing the task to determine if there are team interactions, how the demand will affect the individual(s), and if the workload is too high. Task performance is both dependent on the demand required by the task as well as the skill and capacity of those completing the tasks. The environment *where* the task takes place and the tools and technologies used are often influential in either facilitating or hindering task completion. Analyzing tasks allows all of the variables associated with the different elements of the work system—*who, what, where, when, how, and why*—to be defined and measured. This can guide the design of the work tasks to ensure the demands fit the capacity of the human as supported by the work system.

Designing, creating, and selecting ideal tasks, instrumentation, and required skillsets are difficult endeavors in even less complex work environments like manufacturing. Work design is an element of engineering methods studies that implements and studies tasks and processes to ensure the design of the work and workplace fit the human users. Operative procedures are extremely complex and require continuous efforts to design work through the creation and selection of the best methods, processes, and instrumentation. A comprehensive and systematic procedure to study, assess, and improve work design (tasks and processes) and the work system can lead to ideal conditions for value-based (i.e., safe and high quality) surgery. Yet, work design by itself cannot yield a holistic approach. Instead, by conducting systematic work measurement of the human users, tasks, and other technical and economic factors, standard procedures can be established for tasks to meet needs of the patient, surgeon, and surgical team. As part of continuous improvement, it is critical to explore the tasks, collect and record data pertinent to that process, and to quantitatively attempt to further develop and refine methods. Identifying *who, what, where, when, and how* then continuing to ask *why* is critical to: (1) change the role of the individual performing the task or provide appropriate training to ensure a person with the correct skill level completes the task; (2) eliminate unnecessary, or redesign, unsafe activities to better meet the intended purpose of the task and achieve desired outcomes; (3) replace, remove, or acquire tools and technologies to facilitate the task; (4) change the locations/placement of tasks to better meet surgeon, patient, or staff needs; (5) change the time or sequence of tasks to optimize temporal necessity or personnel resources; and (6) simplify or improve the method of how a task is completed (Fig. 5.1).

There are several methods for analyzing surgical tasks and measuring the task factors. This chapter will describe three common methods utilized in human factors for analysis within the surgical work system and a description of *approaches* within each method (Table 5.1). Additionally, this section contains a description of the outcomes associated with each method (Table 5.2).

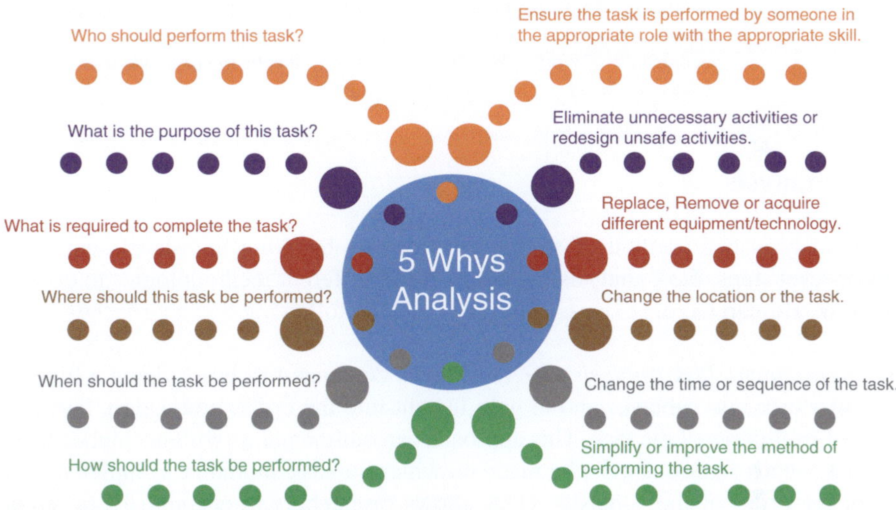

Fig. 5.1 The "who, what, where, when, how, and why's" of task analysis within the surgical work system

Table 5.1 Methods of studying the surgical task

Method	Description	Outcomes
Task analysis	Approaches for breaking down a high-level task into lower-level steps to identify decision points, user goals, and interactions with other elements of the work system	Subtasks, task order, decision points, alternate tasks, goals, motivation
Workload analysis	The measurement of demand required to complete a task to compare user capacity to the task demands to determine fit, safety, and predicted performance	Physical demand, mental demand, performance, capacity, fatigue, burnout
Workflow analysis	A process-based analysis of the time-based flow of tasks, the individuals completing the tasks, and interactions with the environment, tools and technologies, and individuals on the surgical team	Work system interactions, team interactions, task order, efficiencies, inefficiencies, workarounds, patient safety risks

Table 5.2 Outcomes associated with the surgical task

Method	Description	Examples
Patient/ procedural outcomes	Patient outcomes can be associated with completed tasks. In surgery, this is often used to compare techniques, surgical cases with varying complexities and difficulties, and the associated patient outcomes	Length of stay, pain, retained foreign objects, wrong site/ wrong patient surgery, blood loss, Interruptions, operating room ins/outs, quality of life
Surgical team member outcomes	Outcomes associated with surgical team members include the impact of high or low workload due to the demands of the task. The outcomes may be acute or cumulative	Pain, fatigue and discomfort, distraction, quality of life, symptoms of burnout, difficulty
Organizational outcomes	Organizational outcomes will be process measures that impact the business of healthcare. These could include measures of efficiency, resource utilization, and the occurrence of work-related employee injury or illness	Surgical duration, throughput, errors/nonroutine events, reportable evens, workers' compensation requests, staffing levels, material waste

Task Analysis

Task analysis is a method of studying actions by breaking high-level steps into lower-level steps. Task analysis includes several different methodologies to dissect the task. Human factors experts commonly use the following two approaches:

- *Hierarchical Task Analysis (HTA)*—This is conducted to break down a higher-order task into subtasks and to gain insight into the order, motivation, barriers, and facilitators of the task. This approach can outline points within a higher-level task where decisions must be made on which subtask should be completed next or the order of the subtasks. HTA allows researchers to account for different paths in the workflow, which reduce standardization but may allow for autonomy to meet the demands of the surgical case.
- *Cognitive Task Analysis (CTA)*—The approach takes users through steps of a task and inquiries about why each step is taken. These questions get at the motivation or cues that lead to actions. Additionally, researchers gather information on the knowledge and judgment required for the decision-making throughout the task. This approach is often used for developing training guidelines for surgical trainees; however, CTA can help identify the thought process for diagnostics or decision-making when designing decision aids and afford opportunities to improve the surgical team's shared mental model. Through CTA questioning, barriers that lead to workarounds or unsafe actions can be identified.

Workflow Analysis

Analyzing workflow aims to define patterns of work tasks in order to identify opportunities to improve efficiency, standardize tasks, reduce workarounds, redefine roles/responsibilities, and identify barriers or facilitators of successful task completion. Common approaches to complete workflow analysis include the following:

- *Process Map*—This approach maps out the process in a flowchart linking a series of nodes representing the tasks in a process from start to end. The nodes are linked using lines and arrows to show direction and sequence to indicate how and when the steps occur. It is presented in a chronological order; may contain loops in the process, decision points, and roles; and tracks the resources throughout the process. The task could be mapped out as institutional procedures that describe the actions or as the actions take place on a daily basis. This approach can help in identifying tasks that are a part of a workaround that could threaten patient safety.
- *Swim Lane Diagram*—This is a type of flowchart that enables clear distinction of responsibilities across roles. Similar to a process map, the process tasks are mapped out through a series of nodes linked with lines or arrows from beginning to end. However, they are distributed across columns or rows (lanes) to display who is responsible for the different tasks. This approach aids human factors experts in identifying tasks that are conducted simultaneously or are interdependencies where one surgical team member relies on another member accomplishing a portion of the task.
- *Process Failure Modes and Effects Analysis (FMEA)*—This approach is most frequently performed when planning or redesigning a workflow to determine potential for failure. After completing a process map, FMEA can be used to prioritize risks associated with individual tasks. Working with subject matter experts across the healthcare team, these stakeholders identify tasks that include a failure risk. The issues are evaluated and scored with criteria to determine likelihood and severity of occurrence. Then stakeholders work together to create an action plan to manage or mitigate the risk.
- *Time and Motion Studies*—This approach measures the time it takes to complete a series of steps within a task as well as the movements performed by an individual. The timing and movement are observed together in order to identify unnecessary movement or steps within the task and develop engineered solutions to make the work more efficient. This approach emphasizes the importance of the human resource and aims to optimize the system to support the person completing the task.
- *Spaghetti Diagram*—This provides a visualization of the workflow in a work environment. It includes continuous lines tracing the path of an individual or several individuals in a workspace during a task. While it is often used to redesign physical layout of the work environment to support task performance, a spaghetti diagram can also be used to change workflow in order to improve task timing, mitigate congestion of multiple individuals, and reduce workload due to excess movement.

Workload Measurement

Workload is the demand of the task and the associated impact on the person or people performing the task. Workload measurement is required to determine the individual or team resources needed to complete the selected task. There are both subjective and objective measurement approaches. Workload is often measured relative to another task, a different role, or a different step during the overall procedure. For example, workload was compared across surgical roles to determine that the surgeon and surgical resident often have the highest workload across many different workload dimensions [4]. Approaches are often utilized together to more accurately measure workload.

Common approaches to measure workload include the following:

- *Self-Report*—There are several questionnaires for reporting workload. These self-report questionairres include the Rating of Percieved Exertion (RPE) and category-ratio (CR-10) pain scale to assess workload of a surgical task or procedure. One broadly used validated questionnaire to capture workload for surgical team members is the Surgical Task Load Index (SURG-TLX). This is a subjective measurement of physical and cognitive workload as well as four other dimensions of workload in surgery: temporal demand, task complexity, situational stress, and distractions (Fig. 5.2). In this validated survey, users indicate their level of workload on a visual analog scale from 0 to 20 with verbal anchors for each individual dimension [9]. This was used in the above example for both individual and team workload [6, 7].
- *Wearable Instrumentation*—Wearable sensors have become a common approach for measuring physical and cognitive workload during surgical task completion. Physical workload is often measured through muscle activation by electromyography (EMG) and body movement by accelerometers or goniometers. Cognitive workload can be measured through heart rate variability, eye tracking, galvanic skin response, fMRI, and electroencephalography (EEG). This work may occur in the operating room—such as the heart rate variability for measuring workload in the example above [4]—or in surgical simulations as appropriate.
- *Observational Analysis*—Observational analysis, which can be conducted in a variety of ways, includes quantitative (e.g., task time) and qualitative (e.g., near miss) endpoints of interest. Direct observation studies can be completed in person via remote video monitoring and even still photographs. Often these observations can then be used with tools such as the NIOSH Lifting Equation, Rapid Entire Body Assessment (REBA), and the Rapid Upper Limb Assessment (RULA).
- *Cognitive Analysis*—Cognitive, and even emotional, state analysis can be performed again using both quantitative (e.g., eye gaze time for decision making) and qualitative (e.g., self-reported cognitive workload) tools for particular endpoints of interest. The following measures have been readily used to assess the cognitive and emotional workload of surgical tasks and procedures: reaction time, working memory capacity, self-reported mental/cognitive states, task/procedure/technique difficulty, learning curves, distractions, and stress (salivary cortisol levels, heart rate, blood pressure, etc.).
- *Performance*—While intraoperative assessment of surgical performance has mainly been measured during training [10], there are few objective (e.g., time) or

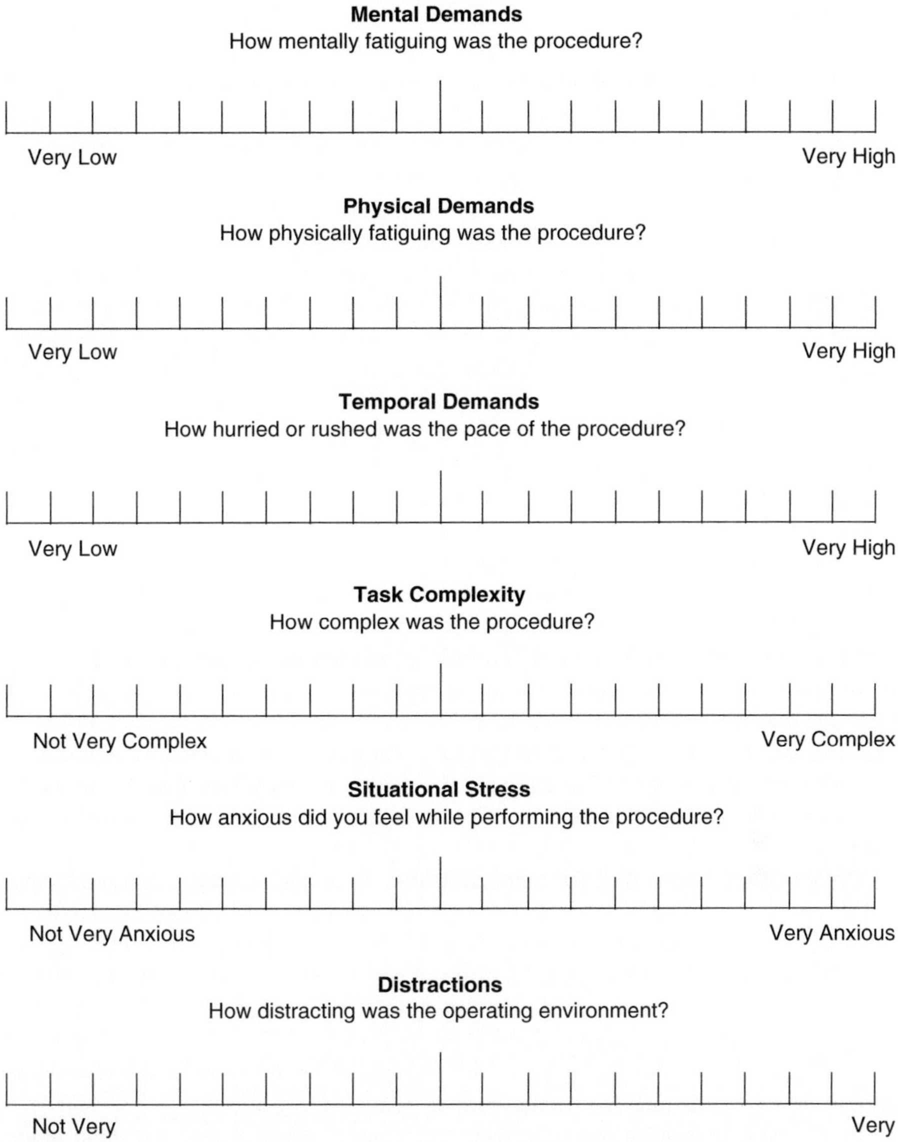

Fig. 5.2 The Surgical Task Load Index (Surg-TLX): A series of six visual analog scales for self-reported surgical workload [1]. (With permission from Wilson et al., 2011; Springer)

subjective measurements (e.g., error rate) of task performance. Didactic surgical trainers have been used for competency assessment and certification within laparoscopic surgery. These trainers have focused on establishing maximum allowed performance times instead of a more traditional approach focused on achievement of average completion times.

Outcome Measures

The outcomes from the analysis of surgical tasks vary and are dependent upon the goal of each method's study. The outcomes may directly or indirectly and impact the patient, the procedures, the surgical team members, and/or the organization (Table 5.2). Most outcomes are comparisons such as using pre-/post-measures during a process improvement study or a comparison to a local or national benchmark.

Procedural measures and patient outcomes already recorded in many operating rooms can provide information on the tasks completed by the surgical team members. Patient outcomes such as length of stay, blood loss, and postoperative pain are commonly collected. In the example above, patient-reported pain was reportedly higher with the novel surgical technique. Since patient care is the ultimate goal of the surgical procedure, these are ideal outcomes for comparing surgical tasks. However, it can be challenging to link a change in the task to patient outcomes. It is often easier to compare procedural differences such as procedural duration or OR turnover times. Larger studies can be statistically powered to detect a change in the number of safety events such as a retained foreign objects.

Beyond the safety of the patient, the surgical team is at risk within the OR. It is well documented that injuries and musculoskeletal illnesses are associated with surgery [3]. During task analysis, reported pain, fatigue, and discomfort can be measured as precursors to injuries or chronic musculoskeletal illness. Work design focused on reducing physical workload, in combination with selection of tools/technologies and environmental changes as a part of the work system, can address a majority of this risk. Self-reported measures on difficulty, distraction, and symptoms of burnout can be used to compare the lasting implications of stressful workload on surgical team members in order to address and prevent work stress and burnout.

Organizational outcomes for a hospital often focus on mortality and morbidity, OR throughput, or readmissions. Analysis of a surgical task could be related to these types of outcomes: commonly, process measures and measures of efficiency are identified as outcomes measures. Identifying opportunities to improve task performance may lead to optimized staffing levels and reduce wasted resources. Additionally, work design may reduce the occurrence of work-related employee injury or illness. Finally, the organization can make strides in reducing reportable patient safety events through sound work design.

In all, the information resulting from analyzing a surgical task will help guide surgical work design and can help improve patient and provider safety and satisfaction while meeting organizational business expectations.

Lessons Learned/Personal Pearls

- Surgical tasks are the actions carried out as a part of the overall work process.
- Surgical tasks vary by surgical team role, procedure type, and patient differences.

- Methods of studying the task include task analysis, workflow analysis, and workload measurement.
- Organizational, surgical team, and patient/procedural outcomes are identified when comparing surgical tasks.

References

1. Kraus TW, Büchler MW, Herfarth C. Relationships between volume, efficiency, and quality in surgery—a delicate balance from managerial perspectives. World J Surg. 2005;29(10):1234–40.
2. McCrory B, LaGrange CA, Hallbeck MS. Quality and safety of minimally invasive surgery: past, present, and future. Biomedi Eng comput Biol. 2014;6:BECB-S10967.
3. Park A, Lee G, Seagull FJ, Meenaghan N, Dexter D. Patients benefit while surgeons suffer: an impending epidemic. J Am Coll Surg. 2010;210(3):306–13.
4. Yu D, Lowndes B, Thiels C, Bingener J, Abdelrahman A, Lyons R, Hallbeck S. Quantifying intraoperative workloads across the surgical team roles: room for better balance? World J Surg. 2016;40(7):1565–74.
5. Bingener J, Skaran P, McConico A, Novotny P, Wettstein P, Sletten DM, Park M, Low P, Sloan J. A double-blinded randomized trial to compare the effectiveness of minimally invasive procedures using patient-reported outcomes. J Am Coll Surg. 2015;221(1):111–21.
6. Abdelrahman AM, Bingener J, Yu D, Lowndes BR, Mohamed A, McConico AL, Hallbeck MS. Impact of single-incision laparoscopic cholecystectomy (SILC) versus conventional laparoscopic cholecystectomy (CLC) procedures on surgeon stress and workload: a randomized controlled trial. Surg Endosc. 2016;30(3):1205–11.
7. Lowndes BR, Abdelrahman AM, Thiels CA, Mohamed AO, McConico AL, Bingener J, Hallbeck MS. Surgical team workload comparison for 4-port and single-port laparoscopic cholecystectomy procedures. Appl Ergon. 2019;78:277–85.
8. Gawande AA, Zinner MJ, Studdert DM, Brennan TA. Analysis of errors reported by surgeons at three teaching hospitals. Surgery. 2003;133(6):614–21.
9. Wilson MR, Poolton JM, Malhotra N, Ngo K, Bright E, Masters RS. Development and validation of a surgical workload measure: the surgery task load index (SURG-TLX). World J Surg. 2011;35(9):1961.
10. Vassiliou MC, Feldman LS, Andrew CG, Bergman S, Leffondré K, Stanbridge D, Fried GM. A global assessment tool for evaluation of intraoperative laparoscopic skills. Am J Surg. 2005;190(1):107–13.

Surgical Performance and the Working Environment

6

Ken R. Catchpole and Myrtede C. Alfred

Case Studies

Example 1: In November 2019, several operating rooms at Seattle Children's Hospital were closed after it was found that 14 patients had been infected, and 6 had died, following exposure to *Aspergillus* mold that was present in the ventilation system. The pattern emerged over several years of routine data monitoring for infections. The eventual response was to install a new air handling system and custom air filters in each room. Routine monitoring of particulate matter and infectious agents within the OR ventilation system is essential.

Example 2: A brand new operating room was being used for robotic surgery on a complex patient, with a new surgical team. As the surgery progressed, the team, unfamiliar with the robot and struggling with the complexity of the case, chose to convert to an open procedure. This substantially added to the duration of the case. As the operation became progressively more difficult and the surgical time extended, the operating room became colder and colder. The surgical team was unable to use patient warming methods – due to the complexity of the case and the failure in the new operating room (OR) to make appropriate equipment available and the patient started to cool down. The anesthesiologist was initially unable to find the controls for the OR temperature, and when they did, was unable to operate it appropriately as it required a technical understanding of the system. The patient became increasing hypothermic over the elongated course of the operation. Moreover, the new OR was several hundred yards from the intensive care unit (ICU), so the transition was longer and more complex than usual, contributing further to patient deterioration and delayed recovery.

K. R. Catchpole · M. C. Alfred (✉)
Clinical Human Factors and Applied Safety Science Unit, Department of Anesthesia and Perioperative Medicine, Medical University of South Carolina, Charleston, SC, USA
e-mail: alfredm@musc.edu

T. N. Cohen et al. (eds.), *Human Factors in Surgery*,
https://doi.org/10.1007/978-3-030-53127-0_6

This demonstrates how people, tasks, teams, technologies, organizational decisions, and the work environment can all interact to create good or bad outcomes. The built environment contributed directly to this incident through poor design of OR controls, lack of appropriate equipment availability, and the distance from the OR to the ICU. This was predisposed by an organizational decision to use a new OR without appropriate consideration for a range of risks associated with new buildings, and became critical when a set of technical problems associated with the surgical approach, technology used, and team, were combined.

The Surgical Work Environment

The physical design, layout, configuration, and acoustic, visual, temperature, humidity and ventilation of each OR and OR suite can influence individual performance, cognition and awareness, teamwork, staff satisfaction, process, infection control, tool and technology use, and thus, ultimately, the success of surgical procedures. As the system of surgery is complex and adaptive, rather than linear and deterministic, the relationship between OR room design and clinical outcomes may not be direct, so traditional clinical evidence is not always available. While there is some evidence relating design decisions to performance, little relates specifically to patient outcomes. Instead, much of what we know comes either from direct observational studies of surgical procedures, or basic experimental work that can be related to measurements in the real world. In this chapter, we explore a range of supposed effects of the built environment on the surgical process, and the methods that can be deployed to understand it.

The Built Environment

The design of every operating suite requires a trade-off among building costs, the size of each OR, and the number of ORs available (See Fig. 6.1). More ORs with a smaller footprint theoretically allow a greater number of surgeries for a reduction in building capital and maintenance but may hamper or even prevent certain types of surgeries. An OR must be large enough to accommodate the patient, team, tools and technologies. While the optimal OR size will differ for different types of procedures, it is generally considered that approximately 400 square feet is reasonable for traditional inpatient procedures. This has steadily increased over time, with 600 square feet recommended for procedures with more staff and/or equipment [5, 7]. This is based on the need for a sterile field and space around it, space for two people to pass each other without touching, and also contains the minimum equipment for a surgical procedure (anesthesia equipment, IV poles and stands, chairs, and waste receptacles). A recent 5-year research project [3, 8–10] – probably the most comprehensive exploration of the range of dimensions associated with safety and performance in OR – identified the following considerations:

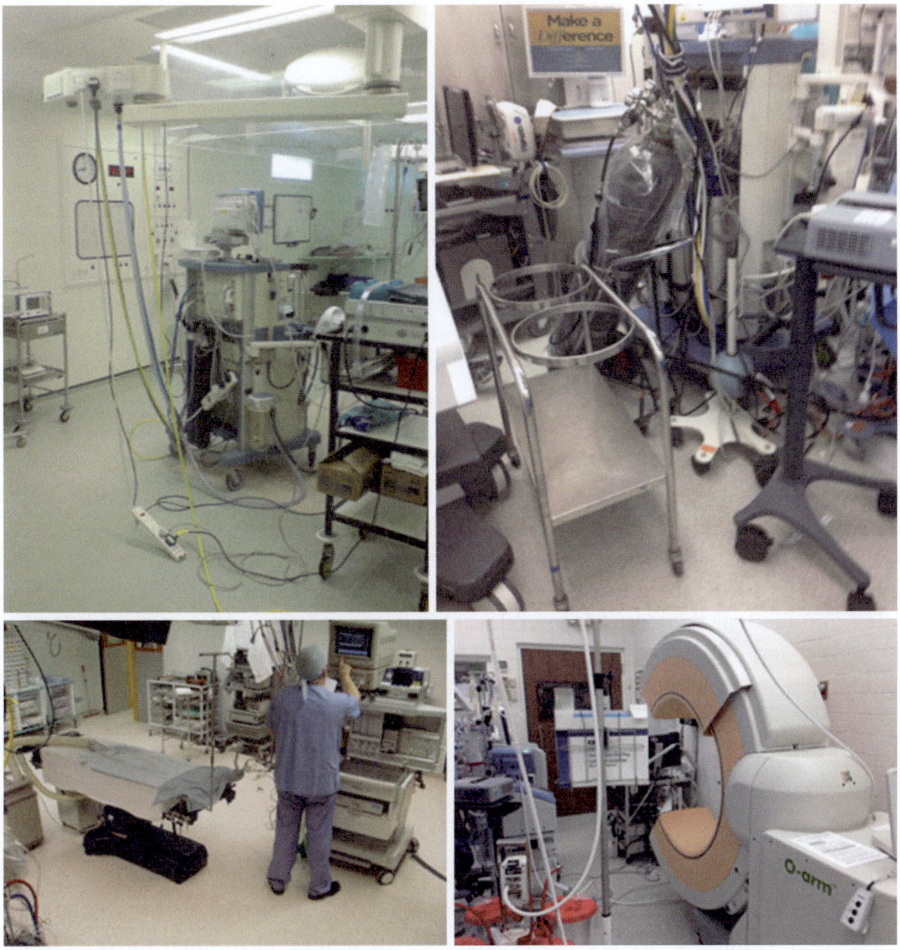

Fig. 6.1 Photos from four different operating rooms in three different hospitals in the UK and USA, showing aspects of space design utilization and common associated problems

(i) Improve movement and flow
(ii) Support visual awareness
(iii) Facilitate digital information access and display
(iv) Reduce disruptions and interruptions
(v) Reduce slips, trips, and falls.

The space needs to be large enough to use for the surgery in question without risk of physical contamination; contaminated airflow; or unwanted interactions between supplies, instruments, or devices. It should provide clear sight lines; facilitate visual interactions and communication among team members; and allow the anesthesiologist, surgeons, and nursing staff to monitor each other. It should have enough space to use, move, store, and maintain a range of equipment necessary for the surgeries conducted within it. It needs to allow easy ingress and egress of people, supplies, patients, beds, and equipment. The floor needs to be smooth, easily cleanable, and sufficiently durable to withstand frequent exposure to a wide array of chemicals and the weight of equipment. Ceiling and wall surfaces should also be easily cleanable and reduce sound reflection. The physical environment should provide enough light for the visual demands of the surgery, permit sufficient light for the rest of the team to conduct their tasks, and allow easy adjustment for different surgical demands. Ideally, the surgical team would also have access to natural light. OR environmental controls should also be available for the team, and electric sockets need to be conveniently located to allow powering of all necessary devices without the cables interfering with the surgical process or movement of people or devices.

The use of an OR suite will change over the lifetime of use, so it needs to be highly adaptable to a range of surgeries and future technologies. Few ORs are designed specifically for certain types of surgeries, as procedures and uses are expected to change over the life of the building. While it is challenging to predict future breakthroughs, we might assume, based on prior developments, that imaging, data, and robotics will be increasingly used, probably requiring more space, more power, improved access to imaging and data displays, and a broader range of display and control devices. Meanwhile, patients are getting older, more medically complex, and larger, so multiple teams may be required, and access to specialized equipment, such as bariatric equipment and lifting capabilities, may also require larger ORs in the future.

The Operating Room Layout

Most ORs can be functionally divided into the "sterile zone," where the surgical procedure takes place and where maintenance of sterile protocol is essential; the circulating zone, outside the sterile zone, which should allow clear movement in, out, and around the sterile zone; and the anesthesia zone, usually at the head of the patient, where anesthesia tasks are completed.

The placement and movement of a variety of equipment, storage, workstations, overhead booms (containing lighting, power, cameras, displays), and furniture (such as tables for surgical equipment, documentation and drug preparation) have to be carefully done so as not to compromise the sterile zone and to allow movement of sterile and non-sterile OR staff around this area. Most of this is the work of the circulating nurse (or nurses), who assists the scrub technician (scrub tech); obtains supplies; configures, operates, or maintains equipment (such as the bovie, or the insufflator and stack in laparoscopy); records the surgical count; and enters data into the electronic health record (EHR). The anesthesiologist or certified registered nurse anesthetist (CRNA) also needs to move about this space, and for specific tasks – such as taking X-rays – other technicians and large devices may be required.

The anesthesia zone has to have enough space for a range of monitoring devices and displays, intubation, ventilation and airway maintenance, and the preparation and delivery of drugs. It also needs enough space for the anesthesiologist and CRNA to work together. Traditionally, the operating table is placed at the center of the room, though this may not always provide the best use of the space. Early studies have suggested that placing the table diagonally in the room can enhance the circulating zone (especially at the foot of the table) while still providing sufficient room for anesthesia.

Multiple studies have demonstrated the surprising frequency with which doors are opened, not just for patient and team ingress and egress, but for procedural reasons (to go for supplies), and for staff to communicate or monitor progress from outside. Sometimes particular ORs are used as through routes by staff to other areas, which does not seem appropriate, but has been predisposed by the design of the OR suite. Frequent door openings contribute to air and surface contamination as well as flow disruptions [9]. OR doors should be positioned to direct the flow of traffic through the circulating zone. Windows can also be incorporated into the OR design to reduce door openings by allowing staff external to the surgery to check on progress visually (or communicate) rather than having to open the door.

There is also the need for multiple storage approaches for a range of basic supplies such as sponges, towels, gloves, gowns (which need to be easily accessible); sterile water, iodine, alcohol solutions, enzymatic solutions; other supplies (such as suction receptacles); and either costly or controlled substances, which are normally stored for charging and dispensing in a controlled, automated cabinet. There also needs to be space for an EHR workstation that will be periodically used throughout the case.

One particular challenge is the location of power cables, which seems relatively simple but can have profound effects for the layout, use, and reconfiguration of the OR space. New technologies and more sophisticated instruments tend to require more space. The introduction of more sophisticated imaging into the OR, such as portable X-ray and CT, image-guided orthopedic and spinal procedural technologies, surgical robots, or interventional catheter procedures, require both space and the ability of the team to work with them while doing a range of other complex procedural tasks. Many of these devices are not assigned to a particular room but are moved in, out, and between as required. This means that not only does the room need to be large enough to accommodate these devices, it also needs to allow paths of access (ingress and egress) for these devices, which are often large. For example, hybrid ORs, allowing for both interventional cardiac catheterization and cardiac surgery, tend to require more space and considerable attention to the location of a range of critical devices, including imaging and perfusion (which may or may not be used concurrently, but in the case of perfusion in particular, need to be quickly accessible).

Ancillary Space and the OR Suite

In Europe, induction rooms are generally used and initially were designed to allow the anesthetization of one patient while another surgery is finishing. Anesthetic rooms provide excellent storage for anesthesia supplies and equipment, and may be particularly popular with patients in general and children especially, but require transfer of the anesthetized patient in the OR, while the original mooted advantage of being able to speed up the anesthesia process cannot be realized, without additional staff. One alternative use for this ancillary space is for equipment breakdown and point-of-use instrument reprocessing post-procedure.

Some OR suites have been designed around the "sterile core" idea, where supplies are located in a controlled environment between operating rooms, but separated from the normal ingress/egress routes for patients. Theoretically, this allows the storage of commonly used items outside the OR (freeing space inside) without increased door openings to acquire supplies, which may compromise sterility.

The surgical process often consists of a preoperative (pre-op) waiting area and a different postoperative(post-op) recovery area. However, many patients, and especially parents of pediatric patients, value returning to the same pre-op waiting room that they left. Ideally, the OR should ideally be located close to post-operative facilities – ether the post-anesthetic care unit (PACU) or the intensive care unit (ICU). This is to facilitate both transfer of patients and to allow the appropriate anesthetic care, which can extend beyond one OR, with anesthesiologists looking after multiple patients for lower complexity cases, and often requiring them to leave the OR to care for unexpectedly sick patients. Physical proximity improves communication and responsiveness.

Ventilation, Temperature, and Humidity

The control of air flow has been seen as vital for reducing infections, with design standards requiring positive pressure differential, downwards from the ceiling (assumed to be cleaner than the floor), with a "screen wall" of air that separates the sterile zone from the outer zones [1]. Together, this aims to push clean air from the ventilation system, down and away from the OR table, and out of the door, thus taking any particulates or potential biohazards away from the patient. However, such "laminar flow" designs may not be especially beneficial for reducing infections, while the regulations do not cover particulate matter to the same rigor as found in some manufacturing environments [15].

Temperature and humidity can also have implications for infections and other organisms. The recommended range is 68–75 °F. for temperature and 40–60% humidity [16]. The appropriate settings need to be balanced with the need to control the temperature of the patient (e.g., in cardiac cases requiring deep hypothermia), and the risks of unintentional hypothermia, which is not infrequent and can have a profound effect on patient outcome. It is a basic requirement to allow control of these environmental settings by the surgical team, but cannot always be assumed. Anecdotally, the difficulty in controlling OR temperature, especially in new, unfamiliar ORs with over-engineered controls, can contribute to hypothermia and catastrophic patient outcomes.

Visual Environment

The visual environment in the OR supports the primary tasks required for success in the procedure; for monitoring of team, patient, and process in support of the primary tasks; and to facilitate beneficial interactions with the outside world.

The basic science of task lighting was conducted in the 1960s and illustrates how tasks requiring varying degrees of visual precision benefit from different levels of lighting [4]. Measured in Lux, boom or head-mounted lighting enables a higher contrast for the surgeon to support the visual precision required. This is particularly critical for fine precision surgery, such as for cardiac and vascular surgery. Allowing a range of motion and multiple light sources on overhead booms also eases movement and reduces shadow effects. Head-based lighting also serves to aid in this purpose. Frequent need to manipulate boom lighting can be distracting, and a number of high technology solutions to help with this have been suggested, but their value has not necessarily been established. For laparoscopy, there is usually a protocol for establishing the appropriate visual environment for the monitor stack, first configuring the white balance, then reducing glare and improving contrast by lowering the ambient lighting in the operating room. This may conflict with other tasks (precision scrub tech work such as counting needles or anesthesia work), so consideration in supporting these tasks might be valuable.

The visual environment also needs to provide visibility of the surgical field and to allow the team to monitor each other. Simple visual cues help team members see when help is needed, or to monitor ongoing activity. An overhead camera helps the rest of the team track the procedure and anticipate requirements without needing verbal confirmation from the surgeon. This is especially helpful for tasks requiring close coordination such as initiation of cardiopulmonary bypass [6]. Similarly, the ability of the surgical team to view anesthesia monitoring can be valuable in situations where shared decision-making is necessary, or where there are significant impacts between surgical and anesthetic tasks.

Windows can allow communication with the rest of the OR suite and offer the potential for some observation. They can also be an important source of natural light, though they need to be controlled during laparoscopic surgeries where contrast needs to be maximized and glare minimized on the surgeon's screen. Placing a window in close proximity to an external scrub sink can also allow the surgeon time to monitor progress of the case preparation while they scrub up and mentally prepare.

As the use of surgical robotics and image-guided surgery has increased, it has presented new opportunities and challenges for the team. Being able to see and manipulate complex visual and monitoring information (such as CT or X-ray imagery) can improve precision of treatments and diagnosis, while the three-dimensional displays on surgical robots provide a perceptual depth unavailable in traditional laparoscopy. However, image-guided surgery requires thoughtful configuration of displays and lighting to avoid glare and maximize contrast while still allowing use of boom and overhead lighting for direct visualization of the surgical field; Even more importantly, the robotic surgery console removes the surgeon from direct physical and visual contact with the rest of the team, necessitating specific communications to and from the surgeon to replace this shared visual environment.

Acoustic Environment

Communication and teamwork are important for a successful surgery. However, many ORs are noisy, impacting communication, creating distractions, and increasing cognitive workload [3, 17]. Sources of noise in an operating room come from ventilation, tools, doors, monitors and alarms, phones and pagers, conversation, and music. Surgical tools, particularly those used in orthopedic cases – saws, hammers, drills – can be especially loud, reaching a peak of 110 dB [11, 14]. It is increasingly being acknowledged that auditory displays on devices – especially warnings and alarms – are also problematic. This presents a number of potential performance-reducing factors related to the acoustic environment [2].

ORs are highly echoic, that is, sound waves bounce off the floors, walls, and multiple other flat surfaces. This impacts speech intelligibility, which is based on auditory localization and sound source segregation [12, 18]. In order to understand what someone is saying, our auditory system filters out the irrelevant signals by comparing the time and amplitude of signals arriving at each ear. It then groups sounds into different "streams" – say, one from someone speaking, one from the music in the corner, and one from the pulse-ox anesthesia sound. We can then direct attention to one or other of those streams to concentrate on that information and exclude others. Stream segregation is a nonconscious process (a good example of how powerful this can be is the "cocktail party" effect, where your attention is drawn to someone from across the room who mentions you, or some other topic of specific interest). In highly echoic environments, auditory signals from a single source bounce around, interfering with signals from the same source arriving directly from the source (sooner) or through multiple reflections (later) and interference with other sources. This makes localization and auditory stream segregation more difficult and consequently lowers speech intelligibility. Thus, theoretically, speech intelligibility in the OR could be improved by putting sound absorbent materials on the walls or ceiling. Though this theory has not been tested, it is supported by observational studies of speech intelligibility, which reduces with increased OR size, and improves with increasing OR contents [13].

The use of music can be controversial. For some, it helps maintain alertness and vigilance and raises the mood of the surgical team. For others, it can be annoying, disruptive and interfere with communications. The science of sound annoyance demonstrates that the perception is not directly related to intensity, but to the implied intent of the source. Thus, rather than necessarily "turning down" music, recognizing that obtaining permission from everyone in the OR to play music, and to agree moments when it might be appropriate to stop it, will help find the right balance for the team.

Human Factors Approaches

The basic human factors approaches to exploring the effect of the OR work environment on the surgical team consist of traditional environmental survey techniques; direct observation; instrumented tracking; and instrumented built environment.

The traditional techniques involve light meters for the visual field (probably measured in Lux). Temperature and humidity can be measured using thermometers and hygrometers. The auditory environment benefits from a range of basic sound intensity measurements (based on the decibel scale, dB), with an added benefit of sound frequency measurement. Usually, an A-weighted network is used, which is designed to reflect human auditory sensitivity (which varies across frequency). Since an acoustic environment will always be changing, the time over which a given intensity is measured is critical. For example, impulse noise (such as a hammer blow) might have a high peak intensity, but may not carry as much overall sound energy or be as disruptive, as a steady-state environmental noise source of moderate intensity. Furthermore, the frequency content of the sound will have an impact on speech intelligibility and other aspects of annoyance.

Direct observation of the surgical team is useful for exploring ingress and egress, movement about the OR, and the potential for disruptions of work from the built environment. A traditional "spaghetti" map can be used to illustrate the usual paths taken by different members of the OR team. This can be complemented with studies of physical interference or disruptions of surgical flow related to the OR layout [3]. Lag-sequence analysis of the passage between two points can also help identify where disruptions, or walking distances, might be reduced by placing equipment or other important items in different parts of the room. Direct observation, eye-tracking, or point-of-view cameras can also be used to explore at where team members look, with a view to facilitating visual scan patterns (much like the "t-scan" in aviation) or reducing spatial interferences.

Finally, a range of other technologies are becoming accurate, available, and affordable for tracking the movement or people and things about an OR and OR suite. Bluetooth, Radio Frequency Identification and other "indoor GPS" technologies can accurately and quickly be used to collect considerable amounts of data on movement. However, they do not replace the need to understand the task or technical requirements that drive movements, requiring care in turning the data that they collect into useable and meaningful information.

Summary

There is no doubt that the design of the OR environment can have a range of effects on individual performance, process, and outcomes in surgery. Basic experimental science exploring how working environments affect human performance is available, which forms the basis for this understanding. However, there remains much speculation and limited evidence about how particular design parameters affect particular processes and patient outcomes. Nevertheless, thinking about how the built environment, the auditory and visual configuration of ORs, and ventilation might be configured to improve surgical performance remains a worthwhile activity. We hope that there will be more opportunities to test configurations and effects in systematic ways in the future.

References

1. ASHRAE. Ventilation of healthcare facilities requirements for surgical suites 2008.
2. Baltin CT, Wilhelm H, Wittland M, Hoelscher AH, Stippel D, Astvatsatourov A. Noise patterns in visceral surgical procedures: analysis of second-by-second dBA data of 599 procedures over the course of one year. Sci Rep. 2020;10(1):3030. https://doi.org/10.1038/s41598-020-59816-4.
3. Bayramzadeh S, Joseph A, San D, Khoshkenar A, Taaffe K, Jafarifiroozabadi R, Neyens DM, RIPCHD.OR Study Group. The impact of operating room layout on circulating nurse's work patterns and flow disruptions: a behavioral mapping study. HERD. 2018;11(3):124–38. https://doi.org/10.1177/1937586717751124.
4. Boyce PR. Illumination. In: Salvendy G, editor. Handbook of human factors. Hoboken: Wiley; 2012.
5. Burlingame B. Operating room requirements for 2014 and beyond. Inside AHSE. 2014 Summer:22–23, 25, 27, 29.
6. Catchpole KR. Task, team and technology integration in the paediatric cardiac operating room. Prog Pediatr Cardiol. 2011;32:85–8. https://doi.org/10.1016/j.ppedcard.2011.10.005.
7. Institute, Facility Guidlines. Guidelines for design and construction of hospitals. 2018.
8. Joseph A. Impact of medical technology on the design of health care settings. Hosp Health Netw. 2008;82(5):suppl 12.
9. Joseph A, Bayramzadeh S, Zamani Z, Rostenberg B. Safety, performance, and satisfaction outcomes in the operating room: a literature review. HERD. 2017;11(2):137–50. https://doi.org/10.1177/1937586717705107.
10. Joseph A, Rashid M. The architecture of safety: hospital design. Curr Opin Crit Care. 2007;13(6):714–9. https://doi.org/10.1097/MCC.0b013e3282f1be6e.
11. Keller S, Tschan F, Semmer NK, Holzer E, Candinas D, Brink M, Beldi G. Noise in the operating room distracts members of the surgical team. An observational study. World J Surg. 2018;42(12):3880–7. https://doi.org/10.1007/s00268-018-4730-7.
12. Leclere T, Lavandier M, Deroche MLD. The intelligibility of speech in a harmonic masker varying in fundamental frequency contour, broadband temporal envelope, and spatial location. Hear Res. 2017;350:1–10. https://doi.org/10.1016/j.heares.2017.03.012.
13. McNeer RR, Bennett CL, Horn DB, Dudaryk R. Factors affecting acoustics and speech intelligibility in the operating room: size matters. Anesth Analg. 2017;124(6):1978–85. https://doi.org/10.1213/ANE.0000000000002118.
14. Peters MP, Feczko PZ, Tsang K, van Rietbergen B, Arts JJ, Emans PJ. Noise exposure in TKA surgery; oscillating tip saw systems vs oscillating blade saw systems. J Arthroplast. 2016;31(12):2773–7. https://doi.org/10.1016/j.arth.2016.05.030.
15. Schreiber K. Rethinking the operating room to prevent surgical site infections. OR Today Magazine. 2012.
16. Van Gaever R, Jacobs VA, Diltoer M, Peeters L, Vanlanduit S. Thermal comfort of the surgical staff in the operating room. Build Environ. 2014;81:37–41. https://doi.org/10.1016/j.buildenv.2014.05.036.

17. Wahr JA, Prager RL, Abernathy JH, Martinez EA, Salas E, Seifert PC, Groom RC, Spiess BD, Searles BE, Sundt TM, Sanchez JA, Shappell SA, Culig MH, Lazzara EH, Fitzgerald DC, Thourani VH, Eghtesady P, Ikonomidis JS, England MR, Sellke FW, Nussmeier NA, American Heart Association Council on Cardiovascular Surgery and Anesthesia, Council on Cardiovascular and Stroke Nursing, and Council on Quality of Care and Outcomes Research. Patient safety in the cardiac operating room: human factors and teamwork: a scientific statement from the American Heart Association. Circulation. 2013;128(10):1139–69. https://doi.org/10.1161/CIR.0b013e3182a38efa.
18. Westermann A, Buchholz JM. The effect of spatial separation in distance on the intelligibility of speech in rooms. J Acoust Soc Am. 2015;137(2):757–67. https://doi.org/10.1121/1.4906581.

7 Organizational Influences and Surgical System Safety

Harry C. Sax

What Role Does the Organization Play in Surgical Safety and Performance?

Medical organizations are reactive by nature – a patient develops a symptom, or routine screening uncovers an abnormality. A series of events flow from the initial finding, additional testing is carried out, and a plan developed. If all goes well, the interventions are effective, and health is maintained or restored. Is it any wonder that that same reactivity becomes central in the investigation of adverse events or the implementation of human factors into solutions? Yet, truly successful organizations have created a proactive culture of "what if?" and have designed programs utilizing the Systems Engineering Initiative for Patient Safety (SEIPS) model in strategic planning or building design. In this chapter, we will examine the organization's role in supporting change and the lessons learned from other industries that have integrated these tools into the culture.

Applying the Concepts in Real Life

I was Chief of Surgery at an affiliated hospital of a large academic medical center. The main institution had several wrong-side surgeries and we responded by establishing checklists and protocols. We thought that we had developed a strong culture of safety. Everyone agreed the knife would not be handed up until checklists were run and the site marked. We were proud to be different than "the Mother Ship."

Then, one of my orthopedic surgeons placed an arthroscope in the wrong knee.

H. C. Sax (✉)
Department of Surgery, Cedars-Sinai Medical Center, Los Angeles, CA, USA
e-mail: Harry.Sax@cshs.org

T. N. Cohen et al. (eds.), *Human Factors in Surgery*,
https://doi.org/10.1007/978-3-030-53127-0_7

The error was not discovered until the patient awoke in the recovery room, and screamed, "My God, they operated on the wrong knee!" The newspapers were calling within hours and my CEO was beside herself with shock and disbelief [1].

What should I do next?

Organizational Influences

Surgery by nature involves risk to both patient and physician. The fact that most cases are completed with little harm is testament to the robust nature of training, team dynamics, technology, and human resilience. Human factors insights are increasingly recognized not just as a part of a root cause analysis, but also as a key aspect of maintaining the health, vigor, and productivity of our providers. The shift in injury patterns in surgeons from back and neck in open surgery to repetitive use in minimally invasive surgery emphasizes the critical need to anticipate the unintended consequences of new technology.

Organizational influences can be broadly categorized into three areas: availability of resources; the operational or "effector" aspect, supporting change management; and the ambiguous term "culture," with its alignment to the basic mission of the entity [2]. There are inherent challenges in each category.

Resource Allocation

Resources come in many forms and the sources of support are often siloed and diffuse. For example, though human capital is controlled by Human Resources, recruitment and retention for physicians are different from those of nurses and support personnel. The influences of unions or the presence of Magnet designation creates different cultural norms in each subgroup and misaligned incentives. Equipment purchases flow through operations, and the value analysis process may focus on how quickly one achieves a return on investment as opposed to whether care will be improved, or the providers' work enhanced. These tensions are being exacerbated by a shift in funding to bundled payments and risk contracts, where investment is seen only as a cost, as opposed to a potential profit center.

Operational Aspects

Once resources are allocated, they need to improve patient care and enhance human performance. Policies and procedures are developed that may not reflect real-world best practices. In well-functioning organizations, the operational leaders have had direct experience "in the trenches," or engage those that do. Multiple strategic initiatives can work at crossed purposes, which becomes especially challenging as organizations expand with mergers and acquisitions.

Organizational Culture

"Mission, Vision, Core Values" are the keynote of an entity's existence. While high reliability organizations (HROs) emphasize safety over funds flow, there will always be a dynamic tension between the two, especially with increased downward pressure on revenues. An increasingly important cultural value is transparency. High-functioning hospitals use their missteps as an opportunity to share and grow. They do not shy away from openly admitting where they have failed. Safety is a primary report at the board level. For example, a list of the names of patients that have been harmed in the previous month is displayed at each board meeting. Culture is on display after an adverse event. How is the science of human factors included in the analysis? Is the response calibrated to the outcome or to the intent of the action that led to it?

Tools and Techniques to Understand Organizational Influences

Using the Human Factors Analysis and Classification System as a Framework to Understand Organizational Influences on Surgery

We previously discussed organizational influences such as resource allocations and operations. The human factors analysis and classification system (HFACS), based on James Reason's Swiss Cheese Model of Accident Causation, can be a helpful framework for thinking about how accidents and errors occur in healthcare. HFACS defines a number of conditions at four tiers: unsafe acts, preconditions for unsafe acts, supervisory factors, and organizational influences (previously discussed) which organizations contribute [3]. This framework can be applied retrospectively on existing data (e.g., event reports or interviews recorded following a serious adverse event) or prospectively during in-situ observations to categorize the types of systemic breakdowns that may contribute to accidents and errors [4]. Perhaps most relevant to our conversation on the organization (outside of organizational factors) is the preconditions for unsafe acts tier – or the tier focused on latent failures that contribute to accidents and incidents. This tier highlights situational, individual, and team factors. Situational factors focus on the physical environment. For example, at a trauma center, multiple resuscitation bays are designed and outfitted to be identical to each other. The team knows the thoracostomy tubes will be to their left and the access trays to the right. Individual factors include the skill sets of the team members and their ability to deliver those skills. This ability changes throughout the day due to stress, fatigue, multitasking, or distraction. Many high-reliability organizations must also provide services 24/7. Normal human diurnal variation, light/dark cycles, and the need to work beyond a normal 8-h shift can lead to chronic fatigue. Further, surgeons are hard driving individuals by nature. They tend to discount their own personal foibles and push limits, which can lead to an unsafe act. Ironically, these same personality characteristics are rewarded by organizations, for example, those that base incentives on relative value units (RVU.) Other vital team factors and skills include leadership, clear communication, and facile coordination among members. Traditionally in medicine, leaders are chosen based on objective measures such as papers published, procedural expertise, or grant funding. These are not necessarily the optimal skill set to lead a team effectively. Additionally, there is increasing interest in the role of Emotional Intelligence in effective surgical leadership [5].

The Categorization of Unsafe Acts

Leaders of an organization must respond effectively to unsafe acts. The key aspect in addressing a poor decision is to categorize it on the degree and intent of conscious actions. Unsafe acts can be broken into violations and errors. Violations occur on a regular basis, often as the workarounds to policies and procedure that do not appear to add value or safety. Many of these evolved over years as a new rule is added in response to a single event. Human nature is to find ways to achieve a task and to avoid specific rules seen as irrelevant. Over time, these actions become part of the culture, a syndrome known as "normalized deviance." By understanding why the work around persists, an organization can either reeducate or alter the process to achieve similar levels of safety without obstruction to flow [6].

On the other hand, there are true acts of commission with willful violation. These include excessive risk taking, disruptive behavior, or practicing above one's level of license. These situations must be investigated with an eye to motivation behind the behavior. Remediation is often indicated.

Errors occur in the subconscious. The individual may not be aware that they are in a situation beyond their skills or training until an accident occurs. Altered sensory inputs such as visual distortions, excessive noise, and flow disruptions prevent relevant information from being processed. When simultaneous processes occur, and priorities may conflict, the practitioner must be able to choose the correct path. This can be aided by mnemonics such as "Airway, Breathing, Circulation" or "Aviate, Navigate, Communicate."

The Just Culture

Marx has published extensively on organizational response to error. He, too, examines the intent of the decision independent of its outcome. If the decision made was found to be inadvertent and unintentional, the response should be similar regardless of the outcome [7].

Similar to the HFACS model, just culture focuses on four actions: human error, negligence, reckless conduct, and intentional rule violations.

Simple human error occurs regularly, often without consequence. We turn left when we meant to go right. We buy 1% milk instead of skim, because we felt we were too busy to write down a list. Diversions and competing priorities are often in play. We tend to recognize this as momentary lapses in judgment or a "Senior Moment." Simple errors in medicine are usually caught by redundancy, but if not, can be the beginning of an error chain.

Negligent conduct suggests a proactive tone. Negligence is a legal definition that includes failure to exercise the significant skill or care expected of the average provider. Negligence reaches criminal levels if the person should have been aware that their actions would cause significant harm. It is basis for justifying reparations. Negligence does not imply a premeditated decision to commit the act.

Reckless conduct is one step above mere negligence. It includes a component of intent and that the person was clearly aware of the deviation yet consciously proceeded. Reckless conduct is associated with a higher degree of culpability than negligence.

Intentional rule violations may or may not be reckless or negligent. Rules or procedures specify a behavior or process. They are designed to standardize procedures and avoid error. In many cases, rules and procedures are created in response to an adverse event. The unintended consequence of excessive rules and regulation is when they are not relevant to everyday operations and therefore are subject to being ignored.

In the just culture scenario, intent is central to organizational response. While it is important to establish clear consequences for negligent or reckless behavior, excessive levels of discipline inhibit open discussion of error, leading to further latent risk. The concept of "the second victim" is recognized as a serious consequence of medical error. Practitioners involved in significant adverse events already are dealing with high levels of guilt and remorse. They begin to second-guess their abilities and the risk for additional harm in subsequent patient care is raised. Add censure by their own organization and it is likely that that a valuable member of the healthcare team could forever be wounded.

Creating a Safe Error Reporting Environment

After a series of fatal accidents, where information was available that could have prevented the incident, aviation created a protected error reporting system. The Aviation Safety Reporting System (ASRS) provides a venue for self-reporting unintentional mistakes that could lead to action by the Federal Aviation Administration. The reports are collated, significant safety trends are identified, and then, they are widely distributed. For example, ambiguity in the wording of an approach clearance brought an aircraft closer to terrain than was intended. After having several reports of near misses, the wording of the approach was clarified. Had pilots who inadvertently committed the error of descending too soon not felt safe reporting, tragedy could have resulted [8]. The culture in medicine is still focused on individual failure. Fortunately, this is beginning to shift, seen by morbidity and mortality conferences now including both human factors and systems in their analysis of the complication.

Organizational Change and Persistence

An organization can embrace human factors to optimize performance; inculcating it into the DNA and engagement by the members is more challenging. Humans do not respond well to change in the short term. Early responses include active and passive resistance or disengagement and underhanded sabotage. With persistent and consistent messaging, change will ensue, albeit at a slow rate. Change is not linear – there is a period of loss with ending of the current scenarios "neutral zone" of the transition and then a new beginning (Fig. 7.1) [9].

Change requires both leadership and management. Leaders must establish direction, motivate, and inspire. They create a compelling vision and are able to support those that follow in this journey. Leaders must work closely with their managers who become the effector arm, as they redeploy resources and set priorities. Problems are dealt with in real time to build confidence in the process and not allow minor setback to derail the process. Stakeholder analysis is key, as the response to each is different (Fig. 7.2).

Kotter breaks down organizational change into eight stages, each with different lengths and strategies to overcome resistance (Fig. 7.3).

The stages range from setting a sense of urgency through eventual consolidation and anchoring the process. This is not accomplished by a single individual as the skill sets are varied. Because the process is long, it is key to celebrate early successes.

The change process itself has key ingredients and various combinations that will lead to success, false starts, or failure (Fig. 7.4) [12].

These ingredients are vision, skills, incentives, resources, and an action plan. Lack of any one of these can move the process in an undesirable direction. These red flags can guide leaders and what is needed to get back on track.

Responding to the Wrong-Side Surgery

We immediately shifted into mitigation mode. We spoke to the patient and their spouse, as well as the operative team. Arrangements were made to assure that treatment of the correct knee was carried out, and support for postoperative recovery

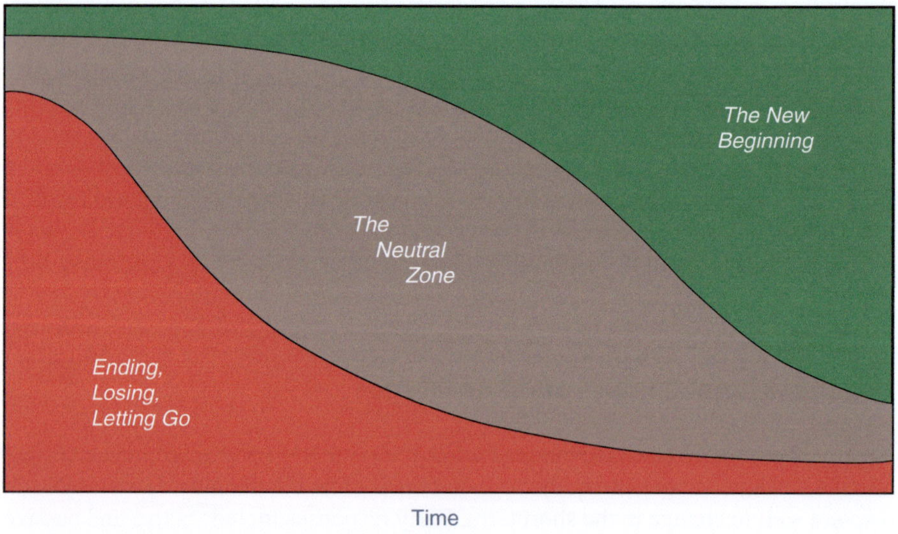

Fig. 7.1 The stages of change. (Adapted from [9])

Fig. 7.2 Stakeholder analysis. (Adapted from [10])

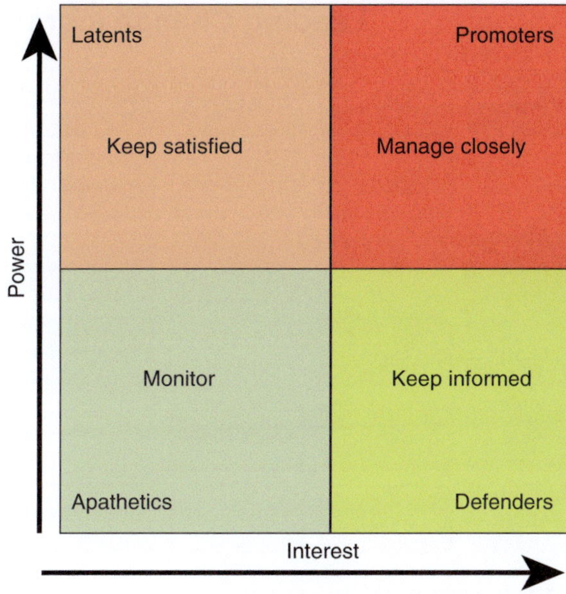

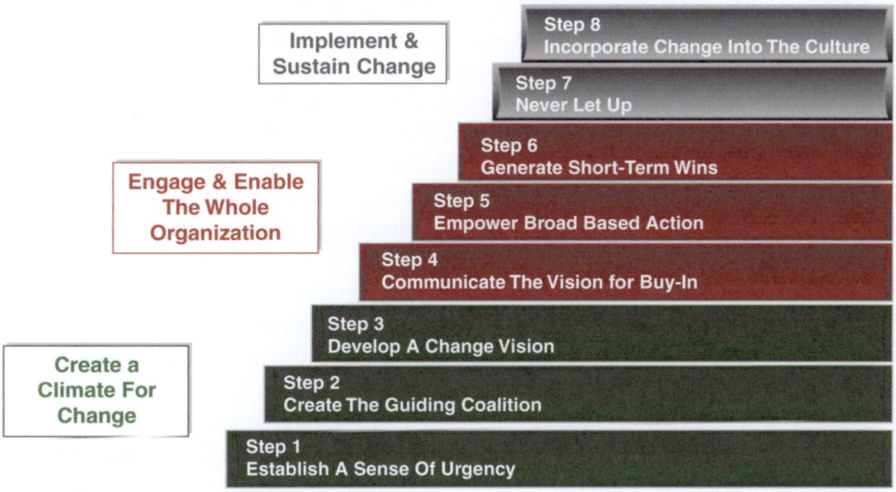

Fig. 7.3 Kotter's eight steps of change. (Ref. 11)

arranged. The fact that the surgeon had an excellent relationship with the patient was a factor in our favor. We notified the Department of Health.

A root cause analysis team was assembled. For unclear reasons, and despite appropriately signing the correct knee, the contralateral limb was prepped and draped. The room had been set up differently, due to equipment availability issues. A resident had placed purple marks on the now draped knee to show scope insertion sites. The checklist was run and on the segment site and side confirmed, team

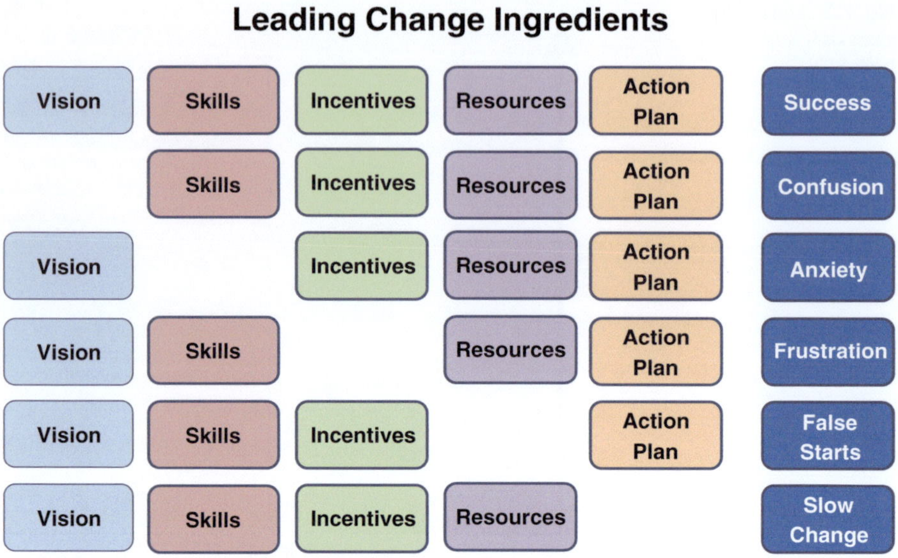

Fig. 7.4 Key components for successful change

members compared the consent and operative schedule. A few glanced at the leg and saw some purple but could not say that they confirmed the surgeon's mark. A traveling nurse was in the room and new to the time-out procedures. She had not been formally oriented as to the procedures. The surgeon was a superb technician but was quick to show displeasure with inefficiencies. Finally, the incorrect knee also had arthritic changes, which is what the physician has expected to see, leading to the delayed recognition of the problem. It was a classic error chain. Issues involving human factors clearly played a role, and I wanted the response to be proportionate to intent of the error.

At a hearing before the State Medical Board, the question before me focused on whether the surgeon, as "captain of the ship," was ultimately responsible. In the past, it was the surgeon who would be censured. I said that we were all responsible, myself included. Because we had been proactive in our safety work, the response was consistent and fair. The Department of Health (DOH) sent a strong message by peer reviewing all members of the surgical team. There was no licensing action, but the findings were made public.

In lieu of formal sanctions, everyone participated actively in fixing the problem, defining the human factors-related issues and more importantly, sharing with others their experiences. Steps in the checklists were clarified. For my part, I led a statewide initiative to standardize the Universal Protocol, and minimize the chance that a surgeon, who might work in multiple hospitals, would have to remember disparate marking and time-out protocols. A patient safety organization was formed to share practices, near misses, and areas of vulnerabilities.

Conclusion

The application of human factors in surgery is not an intellectual concept. An organization must make the decision to do business based on the concept of both human fallibility and motivation, resistance to change, and striving for something better and learning from the past without being restrained by it.

Subsequent chapters put these concepts into action.

Lessons Learned

- Successful organizations create a proactive culture of "what if?" and design programs utilizing the SEIPS model in strategic planning or building design.
- Organizational influences can be broadly categorized into three areas: availability of resources; the operational or "effector" aspect, supporting change management; and the ambiguous term "culture," with its alignment to the basic mission of the entity.
- Violations occur on a regular basis, often as the workarounds to policies and procedures that do not appear to add value or safety.
- Errors occur in the subconscious. The individual may not be aware that they are in a situation beyond their skills or training until an accident occurs.
- While it is important to establish clear consequences for negligent or reckless behavior, excessive levels of discipline inhibit open discussion of error, leading to further latent risk.

References

1. Sax HC. Learning when the Team Fails. In: Gordon S, Feldman DL, Leonard M, editors. The culture and politics of health care work, collaborative caring: stories and reflections on teamwork in health care. Ithaca: Cornell University Press; 2014. p. 119–22.
2. HFACS-RCA Handbook; 2014. Available from: https://www.hfacs-healthcare.com/.
3. Shappell S, Wiegmann D. Applying reason: the human factors analysis and classification system (HFACS). Human Factors and Aerospace Safety. 2001;1:59-86.
4. Cohen TN, Francis SE, Wiegmann DA, Shappell SA, Gewertz BL. Using HFACS-Healthcare to Identify Systemic Vulnerabilities During Surgery. American Journal of Medical Quality. 2018;33(6):614–22.
5. Sax HC, Gewertz BL. Understanding emotional intelligence and its role in leadership. In: Kibbe M, Chen H, editors. Leadership in surgery. Success in academic surgery, vol. 6. Cham: Springer; 2015. p. 67–8.
6. Banja J. The normalization of deviance in healthcare delivery. Bus Horiz. 2010;53(2):139–48.
7. Marx JD. Patient safety and the "Just Culture": a primer for health care executives. New York: Trustees of Columbia University; 2001.

8. Aviation Safety Reporting System. Available from: https://asrs.arc.nasa.gov/.
9. Bridges W. Navigating the Transitions of Change. Available from: http://www.strategies-for-managing-change.com/william-bridges.html.
10. Penn State's College of Earth and Mineral Sciences'. Available from: https://www.e-education.psu.edu/earth107/node/1448.
11. Kotter JP. Leading change: why transformation efforts fail. Boston: Harvard Business Review.; 2007.
12. Jacqueline S. Thousand Richard A. Villa. Managing Complex Change; 2001. Available from: https://my.optimus-education.com/training/teacher-leader-middle-leadership-essentials/managing-change/dimensions-change.

Part III

Broad Surgical Considerations

Human Factors in Perioperative Care

8

Anahat Dhillon, Jessica Lee, and Ashley Fejleh

Introduction/Overview

Despite increasing patient and surgical complexity, perioperative mortality has declined significantly over the past 50 years, especially in developed countries [1]. Advances in patient monitoring and surgical techniques, as well as increased understanding of the nuances of preoperative preparation and postoperative care, contribute to improving outcomes. With an aging population with increasing comorbidities, offering minimally invasive procedures challenges systems and practitioners to continue to maintain high-value care. Focus shifts away from intraoperative outcomes, thereby requiring effective communication between practitioners, increased situational awareness, as well as regard for human error throughout the entire perioperative period. To illustrate human factors principles, we will follow a case through its entire perioperative course.

Preoperative Considerations/Human Factors

Case

A 68-year female with a past medical history of morbid obesity, obstructive sleep apnea (OSA), current smoker, and diabetes mellitus (DM) presents for a robotic-assisted total hysterectomy. Her last echocardiogram showed an ejection fraction of 45% with moderate pulmonary hypertension. In addition, she had poor

A. Dhillon (✉) · A. Fejleh
Department of Anesthesiology, Cedars-Sinai Medical Center, Los Angeles, CA, USA

J. Lee
Critical Care Medicine Anesthesiology, Cedars-Sinai Medical Center, Los Angeles, CA, USA
e-mail: jessica.lee@cshs.org

T. N. Cohen et al. (eds.), *Human Factors in Surgery*,
https://doi.org/10.1007/978-3-030-53127-0_8

exercise tolerance with a Measurement of Exercise Tolerance before Surgery (METS) score of less than four suggesting a high risk for surgery. The anesthesiologist, evaluating the patient on the day of surgery, is concerned about the lack of a stress test. She is also concerned about the impact of insufflation and steep Trendelenburg positioning being associated with inability to ventilate leading to a pulmonary hypertension crisis. There ensues a lengthy discussion with the surgeon about canceling the case and then regarding if proceeding with open surgery is the safest option. The conversation results in anxiety for the patient and a delay in the case.

In a patient-centered multidisciplinary perioperative team model, outcomes require concerted effort; buy-in; and adherence by the surgeon, the anesthesiologist, primary care physicians (PCP), consultants, as well as the patient. As a result, a reliance on communication and coordination leads to multiple points of vulnerability. It has been well established that a visit to a preoperative evaluation clinic decreases day of surgery cancellations, costs related to unnecessary testing, as well as postoperative mortality [3]. From the patient's perspective, a visit may alleviate fears about anesthesia and improve expectations on processes on the day of surgery. Our case example clearly illustrates a patient who would have benefitted from a preoperative workup to further investigate the current severity of her pulmonary hypertension and right heart function. Additionally, she may also be a candidate for pulmonary rehabilitation and risk modification, decreasing her risk of postoperative pulmonary complications, improving wound healing, and reducing the length of stay.

Health care systems must balance the benefits of a preoperative visit with the resource cost to the system, as well as to the individual patient who must take time for a visit. Designing a comprehensive system requires the identification and referral of the patients most likely to benefit with adequate resources and time to allow for optimization and follow up. For example, a patient getting cataract surgery, regardless of comorbidities, is unlikely to benefit and more likely to feel burdened by another visit to a clinic [4]. Conversely, moderate-risk surgical patients may most benefit from a clearance which could be facilitated by a phone call or a protocolized preoperative workup made available to surgical teams and primary care physicians. A select group may most benefit from intensive care coordination and optimization including pulmonary rehabilitation and nutritional support (Fig. 8.1).

In developing the systems for identification, referral, and management of patients preoperatively, each institution should utilize workload and resource analysis to identify the most effective processes (Fig. 8.2). Catchment areas, patient access to clinics, and primary care physicians have to be mapped and overlaid with the existing resources. The utilization of technology such as teleconsultation can further enhance the patient experience and broaden the impact. Human factors design analysis can help streamline the implementation process.

		Surgical Risk Score (SRS)				
Patient Risk Score (PRS)		1 (No Blood loss)	2 (Min invasive)	3 (Mod invasive)	4 (Highly invasive)	5 (ICU care)
	1	Screening	Screening	Screening	Screening	MedClinic
	2	Screening	Screening	MedClinic	MedClinic	MedClinic
	3	MedClinic	MedClinic	MedClinic	APEC	APEC
	4	MedClinic	MedClinic	APEC	APEC	APEC/complex care team
	5	MedClinic	APEC	APEC	APEC/complex care team	APEC/complex care team

Fig. 8.1 Adapted from University of California, Los Angeles complex care team-preoperative risk stratification workup: the most high-risk patients undergoing high-risk surgery and requiring anticipated postoperative ICU care are selected for preoperative optimization and workup

Intraop Emergencies/Incidents

Case

The team decided to proceed with robotic surgery with general anesthesia and an arterial line. Surgery proceeded uneventfully, until the patient experienced a significant sinus pause on ECG followed by extreme tachyarrhythmia associated with unreadable blood pressure on the arterial line. The anesthesiologist initially considered an inaccurate arterial line and spent time trying to "fix" the arterial line. Eventually, the anesthesiologist notified the surgeon and requested immediate desufflation and undocking of the robot and pulse check. The patient was eventually stabilized with vasopressors and antiarrhythmics. Another discussion was held between the surgeon and anesthesiologist regarding aborting the case versus resuming robotically or completing the surgery transvaginally or open.

The Joint Commission identifies communication failures account for 43% of errors in the operating room. Despite its known importance, there are still many

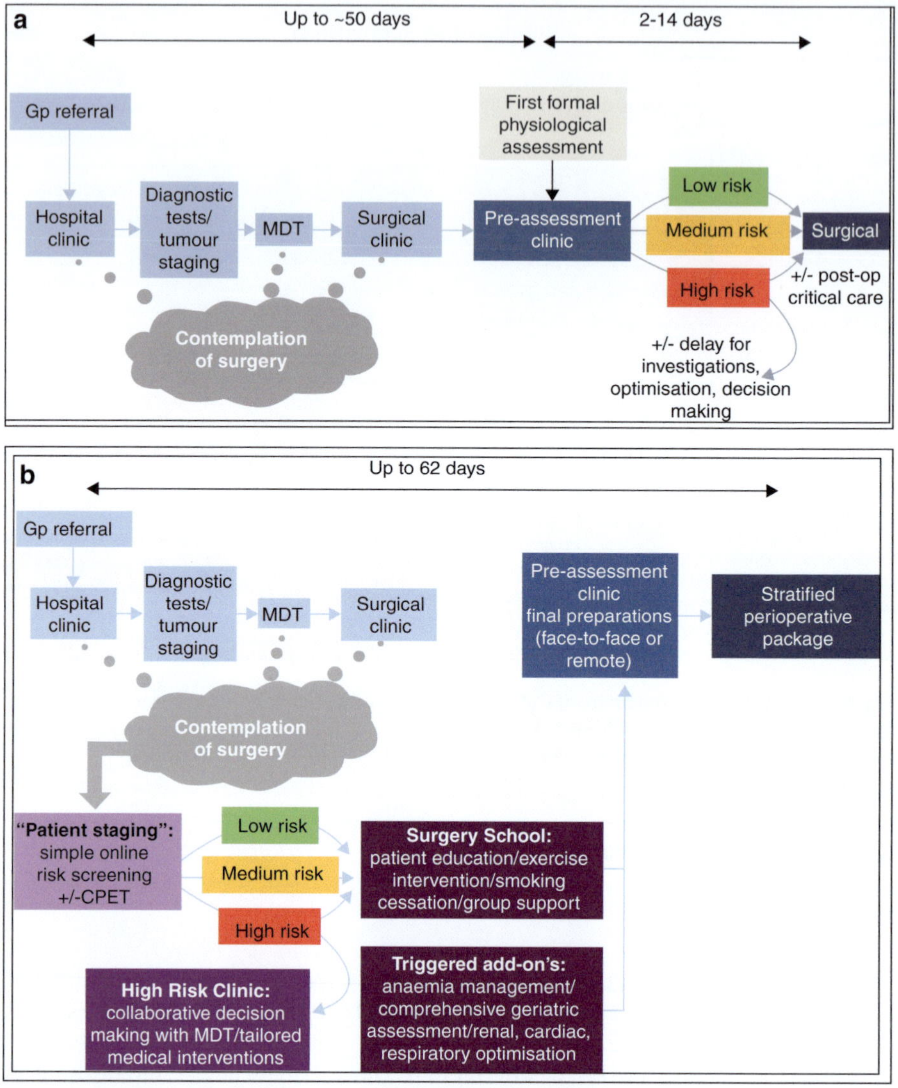

Fig. 8.2 Adapted from Grocott et al. [2] Comparison A. Classic preoperative model vs B. Re-engineered pathway with early preoperative risk stratification and workup/optimization. (MDT: multidisciplinary team)

cases of poor communication during patient care. Why is this and what causes these breakdowns in communication? Identified barriers to communication include poor intraoperative communication skills, fear of how the receiving individual will respond to new or conflicting information, and a lack of closed loop communication. Arguably, the greatest impact on a team performance, like that of the operating room (OR) team, is the leadership dynamic between the surgeon and anesthesiologist within the team.

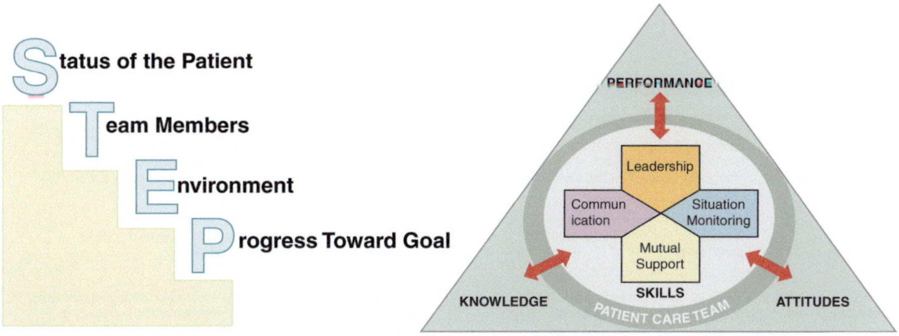

Fig. 8.3 The core principles of TeamSTEPPS (Team Strategies and Tools to Enhance Performance and Patient Safety); four primary trainable teamwork skills are: (1) leadership, (2) communication, (3) situation monitoring, (4) mutual support. These enhance three types of teamwork outcomes – (1) performance, (2) knowledge, (3) attitudes

The use of communication tools is a validated method for reducing medical errors and improving patient care. They range from surgical safety checklists – piloted by WHO and adopted in various forms and implemented in an increasing number of hospitals worldwide; to TeamSTEPPS [6] (Fig. 8.3) – an evidence-based framework used to optimize team communication and performance in health care; and health care handoff tools such as SBAR (Situation, Background, Assessment, Recommendation). Use of these tools intraoperatively has been shown to decrease miscommunication events and foster a culture encouraging team members to voice concern [9].

But do checklists have a role during an *intraoperative emergency?* During emergent situations, even well-trained and experienced practitioners are prone to error, particularly cognitive error, which can be exacerbated by noise pollution (alarms, unnecessary conversations), emotional exhaustion, performance pressure, and fatigue. During a crisis, it is important to understand the prevalence and role of common cognitive errors in anesthesia and surgical settings (Fig. 8.4). The anesthesiologist in our example displays an example of a confirmation bias. In crisis, heuristics assist in time-pressured decision-making, however, inherently exposing clinicians to cognitive errors. Beyond retrospectively identifying these errors, there are tools to mitigate them in real time. The authors use the rule of twos which states that two interventions at two different times not leading to an expected outcome should trigger the clinician to consider a cognitive error.

Cognitive aids reduce decision-based errors and compensate for human fatigue and biases. Comprehensive intraoperative cognitive aids like the Stanford Emergency Manual created by the Stanford Anesthesia Cognitive Aid Group provide anesthesiologists a bright graphic easy-to-read tool [5]. It is designed to guide the user away from fixation errors and confirmation biases through a stepwise approach and differential diagnoses. Likewise, OR crisis checklists such as the one developed between Brigham and Women's Hospital and Harvard School of Public Health have shown improved crisis management in randomized trials in simulated crises.

Cognitive error	Definition	Illustration
Anchoring	Focusing on one issue at the expense of understanding the whole situation	While troubleshooting an alarm on an infusion pump, you are unaware of sudden surgical bleeding and hypotension
Availability bias	Choosing a diagnosis because it is in the forefront of your mind due to an emotionally charged memory of a bad experience	Diagnosing simple bronchospasm as anaphylaxis because you once had a case anaphylaxis that had a very poor outcome
Premature closure	Accepting a diagnosis prematurely, failure to consider reasonable differential of possibilities	Assuming that hypotension in a trauma patient is due to bleeding, and missing the pneumothorax
Confirmation bias	Seeking or acknowledging only information that confirms the desired or suspected diagnosis	Repeatedly cycling an arterial pressure cuff, changing cuff sizes, and locations, because you 'do not believe' the low reading
Framing effect	Subsequent thinking is swayed by leading aspects of initial presentation	After being told by a colleague, 'this patient was extremely anxious preoperatively', you attribute postoperative agitation to her personality rather than low blood sugar
Commission bias	Tendency toward action rather than inacton. Performing un-indicated manoeuvres deviating from protocol. May be due to overconfidence, desperation, or pressure from others	'Better safe than sorry' insertion of additional unnecessary invasive monitors or access; potentially resulting in a complication
Overconfidence bias	Inappropriate boldness, not recognizing the need for help, tendency to believe we are infallible	Delay in calling for help when you have trouble intubating, because you are sure you will eventually succeed
Omission bias	Hesitation to start emergency maneuvers for fear of being wrong or causing harm, tendency towards inaction	Delay in calling for chest tube placements when you suspect a pneumothorax, because you may be wrong and you will be responsible for that procedure
Sunk costs	Unwillingness to let go of a failing diagnosis or decision, especially if much time/resources have already been allocated. Ego may play a role	Having decided that a patient needs an awake fibreoptic intubation, refusing to consider alternative plans despite multiple unsuccessful attempts
Zebra retreat	Rare diagnosis figures prominently among possibilities, but physician is hesitant to pursue it	Try to 'explain away' hypercarbia when MH should be considered
Unpacking principle	Failure to elicit all relevant information, especially during transfer of care	Omission of key test result, medical history, or surgical event

Fig. 8.4 Examples of common cognitive errors in anesthesia, with examples. (Adapted from Stiegler et al. [10])

Postoperative Care

Case

A decision was made to complete the surgery transvaginally as it was agreed that the patient was too unstable for robotic surgery and too late to abort the case as the uterus had already been devascularized. The patient was stabilized and extubated in the operating room. The surgeon requested admission to the inpatient floor; however, the anesthesiologist recommended postoperative ICU monitoring.

Postoperative care including initial disposition and timely identification of any postoperative complications is an extremely important element of the perioperative period that can define the patient's overall course. Unforeseen postoperative complications delay length of stay, resource utilization, and contribute to patient mortality and morbidity [7]. Elements of the postoperative period that are prone to human factors include disposition planning thorough handoff between care teams, attention and management of patient's comorbidities, and implementing Enhanced Recovery After Surgery (ERAS) protocols where appropriate.

In deciding the right place for a patient, preoperative care coordination can significantly impact outcomes by ensuring that high-risk patients are considered for an appropriate level of postoperative monitoring. Postoperative patients transferred from the floor to the ICU have worse outcomes than those admitted directly to an ICU or those never transferred back. Although not specifically proven, it seems likely that a high-risk patient admitted to the ICU for monitoring is less likely to suffer a complication and thereby have improved outcomes and decreased length of stay. Preoperative planning for disposition allows the health system to better estimate patient bed flow. Additionally, team dynamics in the operating room as well as good communication ensure perspectives of all team members are considered in determining appropriate care.

Transfer of care occurs frequently and across disciplines throughout the perioperative period. Each exchange of information about the patient introduces the possibility of communication error which can jeopardize patient safety. For this reason, the Joint Commission requires "a standardized approach" for handoffs to minimize adverse events. A proper handoff to the post-anesthesia care unit or the ICU should include all providers involved in the case including OR nurses, surgical team, anesthesia team. Not only is it important to provide a thorough handoff, it is also important the information is received. For this reason, some institutions require a pause for patient identification with handoff when all teams are present and attentive. Even if handoffs are standardized, it is important to recognize there can still be variable quality and quantity of information exchanged. Succinct or protocolized checklist expedites the handoff process while maximizing the quality of the information provided (Fig. 8.5) and resulting in improved outcomes [8].

In the postoperative period, measures for accelerated recovery include early mobilization, pulmonary hygiene, physical therapy/occupational therapy, adequate nutrition, preventing pressure ulcers/skin integrity, and pain control as part of ERAS protocols decrease length of stay. While many patients qualify for these protocols across surgical specialties, systems to identify patients that are not appropriate preoperatively as well as systems for early rescue of complications are necessary to ensure patient safety.

Patient	Patient Identification (Nameband check)	
	Time In	
	Allergies	
	Surgical Procedure and Reason for Surgery	
	Type of Anesthesia (GA, TIVA, regional)	
	Surgical or anesthesia complications	
	PMH and ASA Scoring	
	Preoperative Cognitive Function	
	Preoperative Activity Level (METs)	
	Limb Restriction	
	Preop Vitals	
Procedure	Positioning of Patient (if other than supine)	
	Intubation conditions (grade of view, airway, quality of bag mask ventilation, bite block?)	
	Lines/catheters (IVs, a-lines CVSs, foley chest tubes, surgical drains, VP shunt)	
	Fluid Management	Fluid= EBL= UO=
Medications	Analgesia Plan - During Case, Postop Orders	
	Antiemetics Administered	
	Medications due during PACU (antibiotics, etc.)	
	Other Intra-OP Medications (steroids, antihypertensives)	

"Do you have any questions or concerns?"

Fig. 8.5 Example of handoff checklist used at Georgetown University Hospital. (https://www.apsf.org/article/improving-post-anesthesia-care-unit-pacu-handoff-by-implementing-a-succinct-checklist/)

Conclusion/Pearls/Things We Learned

- Human factors play a significant role in patient safety and outcomes in the perioperative period.
- Preoperative patient risk stratification allows for more efficient use of resources and improved medical optimization prior to surgery.
- Communication is key to safe patient care: use of intraoperative and hand-off communication tools decreases miscommunication events and fosters a culture encouraging team members to voice concern.
- Cognitive aids reduce decision-based errors and compensate for human fatigue and biases.
- Appropriate preoperative care coordination also addresses postoperative disposition, resulting in decreased complications and shorter length of stay.
- By recognizing potential errors, practicing effective communication, and utilizing available cognitive aids/tools, perioperative medicine can reduce adverse events.

References

1. Bainbridge D, Martin J, Arango M, Cheng D, Evidence-based Perioperative Clinical Outcomes Research (EPiCOR) Group. Perioperative and anaesthetic-related mortality in developed and developing countries: a systematic review and meta analysis. Lancet. 2012;380:1075–81.
2. Grocott MPW, Plumb JO, Edwards M, et al. Re-designing the pathway to surgery: better care and added value. Perioper Med. 2017;6:9.
3. Jeanna D, Blitz MD, Samir M, Kendale MD. Preoperative evaluation clinic visit is associated with decreased risk of in-hospital postoperative mortality. Anesthesiology. 2016;125:280–94.
4. Chen C, Lin G, Bardach N, et al. Preoperative medical testing in medicare patients undergoing cataract surgery. N Engl J Med. 2015;372:1530–8.
5. Howard SK, Chu LK, GoldhaberFiebert SN, Gaba DM, Harrison TK, Stanford Anesthesia Cognitive Aid Group. Emergency manual: cognitive aids for perioperative clinical events. See http://emergencymanual.stanford.edu for latest version. Creative Commons BY-NC-ND. 2013 (creative commons.org/licenses/by-nc-nd/3.0/legalcode).
6. Weld LR, Stringer MT, Ebertowski JS, et al. TeamSTEPPS improves operating room efficiency and patient safety. Am J Med Qual. 2016 Sep;31(5):408–14. https://doi.org/10.1177/1062860615583671.
7. Jones CPL, Fawker-Corbett J, Groom P, et al. Human factors in preventing complications in anaesthesia: a systematic review. Anaesthesia. 2018;73(Suppl 1):12–24.
8. Arora V, Johnson J. A model for building a standardized hand-off protocol. Jt Comm J Qual Patient Saf. 2006;32:646–55.
9. Arriaga A, Bader A, Wong J, et al. Simulation-based trial of surgical-crisis checklists. N Engl J Med. 2013;368:246–53.
10. Stiegler MP, Neelankavil JP, Canales C, Dhillon A. Cognitive errors detected in anaesthesiology: a literature review and pilot study. BJA. 2012;108(2):229–35.

Counting Backwards: Tracing the Effect of Human Factors in Anesthesiology

9

Kristen L. W. Webster and James H. Abernathy

What Is Anesthesiology

During procedures, anesthesiology providers are responsible for ensuring patient unconsciousness, providing appropriate pain relief, optimizing patient surgical conditions, ensuring optimal perfusion of all organ systems, and preparing the patient for an expedited and enhanced recovery.

Case Study

A 79-year-old 103 kg female with newly diagnosed pancreatic cancer presented to the operating room (OR) for a Whipple procedure. At the Amazing Hospital, anesthesiologists practiced alone in the operating room. Preoperative workup and risk factor modification were unremarkable. An epidural was placed preoperatively. The patient was induced with standard medications, intubated, and appropriate intravenous (IV) access and arterial monitoring were placed. About an hour into the case, while the surgeon was dissecting around the portal vein, the blood loss began; it was not a dramatic blood loss, but it was more insidious and steady. The anesthesiologist reflexively increased the rate of IV fluid administration, and the noise from the suction continued. But the anesthesiologist was unaware of the amount of blood loss because the collection canister was hidden on the other side of the boom, out of sight. Forty-five minutes later, the patient's heart rate had increased 20% above

K. L. W. Webster
Department of Process Improvement, University of Louisville Health, Louisville, KY, USA

J. H. Abernathy (✉)
Department of Anesthesiology and Critical Care Medicine, Johns Hopkins University, Baltimore, MD, USA
e-mail: jaberna4@jhmi.edu

T. N. Cohen et al. (eds.), *Human Factors in Surgery*,
https://doi.org/10.1007/978-3-030-53127-0_9

baseline, and her blood pressure was about 20% less, neither remarkable in their values but both suggesting hypovolemia.

A second anesthesiologist came in to offer the first anesthesiologist a break. A perfunctory handoff occurred. Concern for blood loss was not addressed in the handoff. While the primary and first anesthesiologist was out on break, the patient's blood loss quickened, and the patient arrested. Cardiopulmonary resuscitation (CPR) and advanced cardiac life support (ACLS) ensued. Emergency release blood was given along with resuscitation medications, and the patient's blood pressure returned to normal. After adequate resuscitation, the patient did well and was discharged home after staying about a week in the hospital.

Post analysis of the event revealed an operating room where the music was loud, communication was delayed due to misunderstanding and inability to hear over music in the OR, suction canisters were placed out of sight of the anesthesiologists, and the nursing team did not feel empowered to speak up.

How Can We Improve Anesthesiology Using Human Factor Principles?

The anesthesiologist, commonly relegated to the head of the patient, is surrounded by towering machinery and separated from the surgical field by a sterile drape. Monitors display the patient's vital signs, ventilator parameters, and depth of anesthesia. These variables cycle at varying intervals, and alarms sound with varying intensity. Monitoring the incredible amounts of information created during surgery requires high levels of vigilance and interactions with the multiple pieces of equipment. Yet, the physical and cognitive environments are rarely considered when creating the structures, machines, and tools necessary for anesthesiologists to complete their jobs. This chapter will expand upon numerous shortcomings in the design of the anesthesiologist's workspace and offer insights to improvement through application of human factors principles.

Physical Ergonomics

Anesthesiologists must accommodate to other providers' work fields, while keeping their own sterile. At the head of the bed, anesthesiologists are visually confined to their space while monitoring fluid levels and gas saturation levels. Drapes, wires, and machinery can obscure other visual cues that may trigger immediate response, like blood loss. Further, these obstacles can cover access points like intravenous or central lines and other items like suction canisters. These obstacles require that the anesthesiologist maneuver within the workspace, bending, twisting, and contorting to see or interact with the lines (See Fig. 9.1). While this is a common workflow, it can lead to serious repercussions to the musculoskeletal system.

Work-related musculoskeletal disorders (WRMSDs) are commonly associated with or caused by repetitive, continuous or high-force motions, and/or misalignment

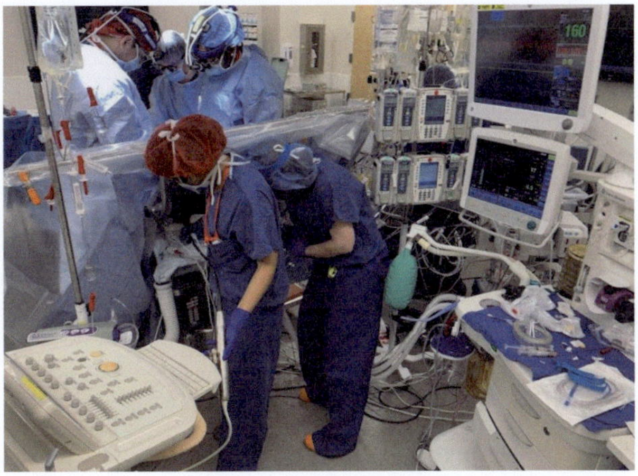

Fig. 9.1 Anesthesiologist and resident strain to reach under the sterile drape

of the body during action [1]. WRMSDs can cause muscle fatigue, pain, injury, and illness, resulting in the loss of work time due to recovery or the inability to perform certain functions. As a result, this leads to decreased job satisfaction and work performance [2]. While many organizations address these issues by providing sessions supporting relaxation techniques, medication, and exercise opportunities [3], a more sustaining approach to reducing WRMSDs would be preventative through user-centered designs.

Anesthesiologists receive little attention in the literature regarding the discomfort associated with the job. Because the operating table is placed in regard to the needs of the surgeon, anesthesiologists must maneuver under opaque drapes, through lines, while generally bent over in order to administer medications. Low operating table heights have been referenced as reasons for pain in regard to administering spinal anesthesia, but this discomfort would persist with any low table arrangement such as the operating table [4]. The operating table is generally placed as needed for the operating surgeon, commonly low or in a position that allows optimal access to the surgical site. While this is necessary and vital for patient safety and to protect the musculoskeletal structure of the surgeon, this often means that other providers such as the anesthesiologist (or perfusionist) must consistently adjust their own body positions and workflow to accommodate for the surgeon's preferred table height or the necessary position of the table for that particular surgery. Placement of equipment requires anesthesiologists to choose between visualizing the equipment or their physical comfort and safety. This could potentially be avoided by introducing the ability to adjust the height of the provider rather than the height of the operating room. This can be accomplished with stools, ramped operating room floors, or recessed floor spaces for anesthesia providers.

Tubes, wires, and cables can lead to workplace injury due to slips, trips, and falls [5]. To prevent providers from injuring themselves, electrical and mechanical connection design should take advantage of the vertical space in the OR by attaching to ceiling-mounted booms. Gas flow to anesthesia equipment would greatly benefit from this vertical orientation. When not able to accommodate for a vertical

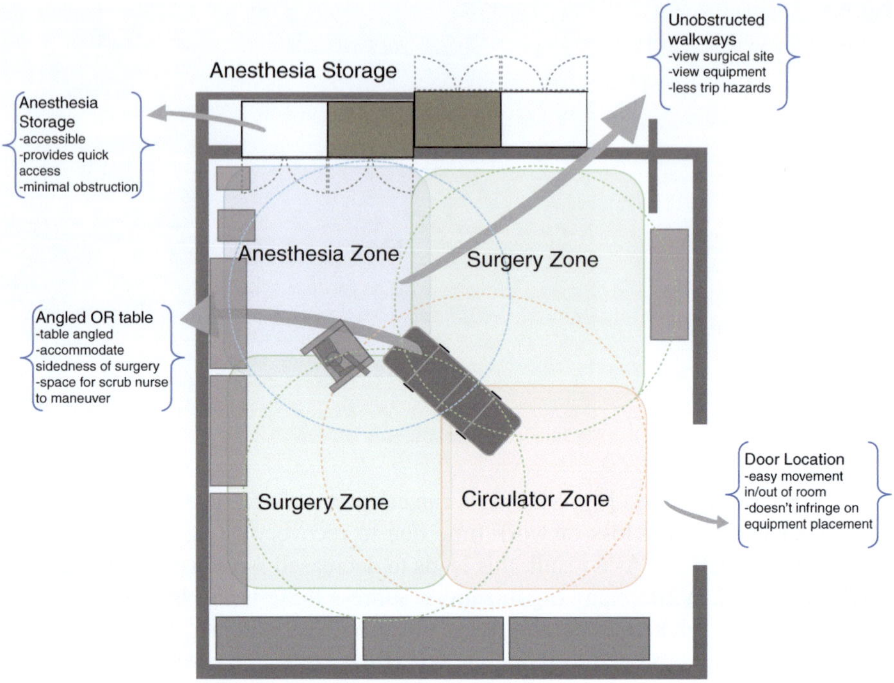

Fig. 9.2 Suggested layout for anesthesia space

orientation, rubber mats should be used to reduce the risk of fall by covering exposed cables and wires. Further, the extension of these cables and wires can be reduced by designing the surgical bed as the main power hub, so that electrical power, gases, and light sources radiate outward from the operating table rather than the exterior of the room [6].

OR designs could greatly benefit from the influence of human factors engineering principles. Previous iterative design processes have recommended that OR beds be angled. (See Fig. 9.2). This places the anesthesia workstation away from the door, minimizing interruptions caused by others passing through the anesthesia workspace. Additionally, this arrangement allows anesthesia personnel to maximize the use of space in the OR and providing more accommodation for storage space. Other considerations in this design include the need for a hardwired phone and a wall-mounted glove dispenser [7].

Cognitive Support

The anesthesia workspace requires revision not only to improve physical conditions but to support cognitive conditions as well.

The operating room can reach deafening levels, up to 80 dB and higher, which can inhibit expedient and necessary communication when coordinating medical care, especially during emergent situations. These decibel levels sometimes exceed the Occupational Safety and Health Administration and National Institute of Occupational Safety and Health standards [8, 9]. Noise pollution in the OR comes from many sources, including general conversations, general practices in the OR generated from work tasks (i.e., typing, exchanging surgical tools, equipment operation), music, and alarms being a frequent contributor.

Within any procedure, an average of 1.2 alarms takes place per minute, of which approximately 80% are deemed to have no therapeutic consequences [10], requiring the anesthesiologist to decide at least once a minute if action must be taken, demanding the anesthesiologist be at a constant state of arousal and vigilance. Or, worse, creating an atmosphere where the anesthesiologist ignores all alarms. As demonstrated through signal detection theory (Fig. 9.3), this type of environment leads to increased desensitization of the observer due to the number of false positives, meaning that it is less likely for a correct identification of an alarm that requires action. These cognitive and physical barriers, or flow disruptions, as they are commonly called, are correlated with higher perceived workloads, higher stress levels, and potential negative patient outcomes and length of surgery [11]. To address this issue, suggestions have been made to require calibration specific to each patient, integration of algorithms that analyze the whole system, increase sensitivity in the measurement, and that equipment manufacturers provide different signals or tones for alarms based on the priority of response needed. Tones could vary by pitch, loudness, or cadence.

Because the operating room environment demands that anesthesiologists switch between tasks every 9 seconds—communicating with other providers, managing anesthetic levels and other vitals, drawing up medications, and other tasks—it is important to limit the need to preform higher cognitive functions such as computing calculations [12]. The literature has demonstrated the inability for humans to multitask and instead rapidly task-switch. This work highlights the need to condense complex information within the visual displays to support the ability for the anesthesiologist to focus on the direct needs of the patient and less on maintenance of the equipment, such as false alarms, electronic medical record entry, or data, which do not directly affect the safety of the patient.

The anesthesia workspace requires that the provider balance information from others as well as complex machinery and, as such, can be regarded as a

Fig. 9.3 Signal and response outcomes

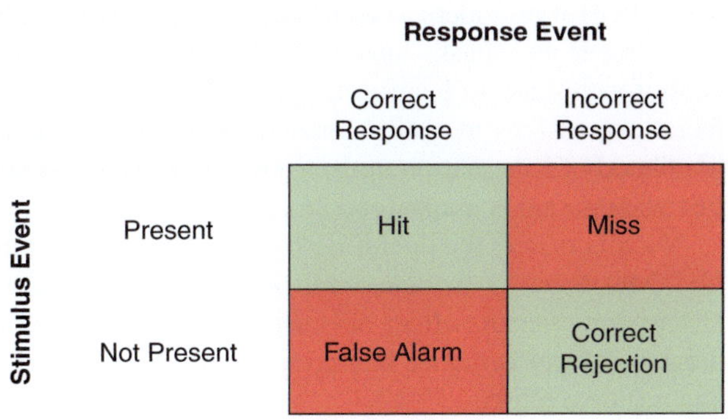

human–machine–system. This system is "information-intensive" and places a large mental load upon the anesthesiologist [13]. Designing anesthesia equipment, machinery, and software with the user in mind can assist in relieving mental load, physical strain, and communication errors.

Communication

As a foundation for all interactions with a team, communication is paramount for high-reliability performance. As a high-risk, high-consequence environment, the operating room depends upon effective teamwork and reliable communication channels.

It is difficult for the anesthesiologist to obtain all the possible patient information perioperatively. The timing of surgeries and requirements for documentation and consent signing often means that the anesthesiologist is provided time for a brief conversation with the patient to sign consents and ensure the correct procedure is being followed, then a handoff with the pre-op nurse before wheeling the patient back to the operating suite to prepare and place the patient under anesthesia. This type of short communication style trends throughout the whole surgery.

Anesthesiologists are provided short breaks to eat, check on other patients, or step out of the operating room for other reasons. This break requires that the anesthesiologist hand off the patient to an incoming anesthesiologist delivering critical and timely information as quickly as possible without decreasing the level of vigilance. Handoffs have been criticized within the literature for the lack of ability to pass all pertinent information in a reasonable amount of time. Further, handoffs increase the risk of controlled drug discrepancies [14]. This highlights the need to reduce the amount of transfers of care during anesthesia and the need for standardized hand-off protocols. Though structured conversations are awkward for the users, highly structured conversations can potentially reduce noise clutter and improve communication [15].

Guttman et al. posits an updated model (Fig. 9.4) of communication that acknowledges that attitudes, behaviors, and cognitions (ABCs) are influenced by internal and external factors [16]. These barriers can be overcome by increasing the use of closed-looped communication techniques such as "check backs," clarification, assurance of accuracy, and precision. Additionally, the environment can be changed to support the ability for providers to communicate visually as well as auditorily. For example, clear drapes and masks have been demonstrated to improve communication, especially for those with hearing loss [17, 18]. The ability to see the full face and read facial expressions as well as watch the mouth of the active speaker increases the likelihood of information transmission between the two parties. Check backs ensure that what is said is understood and assists in limiting miscommunications.

Not all noise in the operating room is created by equipment, alarms, or conversation. Music can contribute a considerable amount of noise in the operating room. Discussion over the effect of music on surgeon performance, communication, and mental task performance has been varied, with studies suggesting positive, neutral, and negative effects.

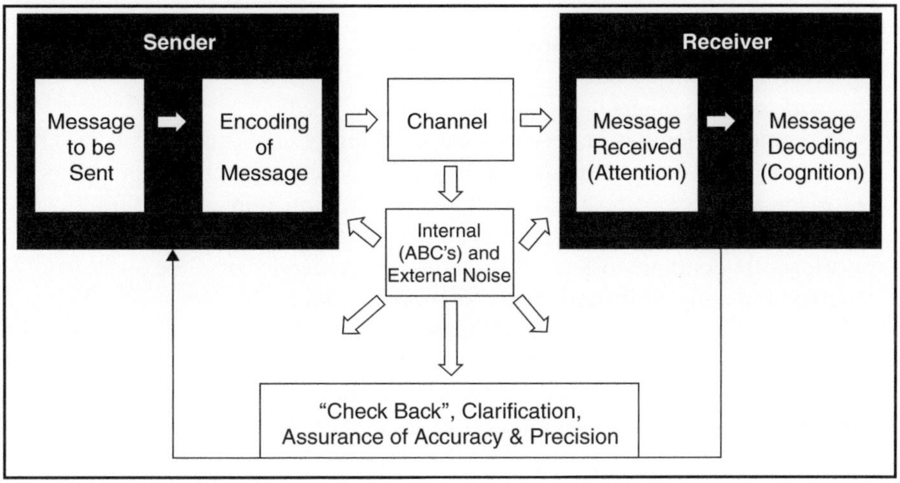

Fig. 9.4 Communication model in healthcare. (Adapted from Guttman et al. [16])

The effects of music on anesthesiologists are still unknown. Overall, 26% of anesthesiologists felt that vigilance and communication was negatively affected by music, and 51% believed that music was distracting when resolving a problem [19]. Yet other studies are unable to demonstrate a link between music and psychomotor testing like vigilance, tack, and reaction time in anesthesia residents [20].

Compounding Issues

The design of the workspace is a compounding and cascading issue. In particular, human factors offer the ability to evaluate systems as a whole and place the user as the focal point. Placement of the anesthesiologist as the focal point within their workspace highlights how sub-optimal conditions can radiate to affect not only the patient but also the other healthcare providers in the operating room. As referenced earlier, an unacceptable loss of blood should trigger an immediate response, but then the blood detection device is obscured by a boom and consistently out of reach and sight of the anesthesiologist; the ability to detect the loss of blood and, subsequently, time to react to this blood loss is increased. Without the ability to detect the blood loss, the anesthesiologist is unable to communicate this to the surgeon who may or may not realize the accumulation of blood loss. Items like this demonstrate the need for accurate and precise redundancy measures. Rather than relying on visual inspection or estimations, collection tools should provide accurate weights and alarm when a pre-programed weight has been reached. As discussed previously, these alarms should be calibrated precisely for each patient to reduce false alarms and potentially have unique tones or audible/visual signals to allow the providers to distinguish them from other alarms.

Lessons Learned/Personal Pearls

- Redesign of the anesthesia workspace while determining the effects of the workspace on others in the operating room is needed.
- Communication has largely focused on auditory confirmation, but visual feedback can be used to improve information exchange between providers.
- Medical device companies need to do a better job at integrating frontline user insights and human factors professionals to improve the device design.
- Handoffs continue to require research and development to be successful and limit communication failure–associated harm.

References

1. National Research Council and the Institute of Medicine. Musculoskeletal disorders and the workplace: low back and upper extremities. Panel on musculoskeletal disorders and the workplace. Washington, DC: National Academy Press; 2001.
2. Evanoff BA, Bohr PC, Wolf LD. Effects of a participatory ergonomics team among hospital orderlies. Am J Ind Med. 1999;35(4):358–65.
3. Cartwright S, Cooper C, Murphy L. Diagnosing a health organization: a proactive approach to stress in the workplace. In: Job stress interventions. Washington, DC: American Psychological Association; 1995. p. 217–33.
4. Sohn H-M, Kim H, Hong J-P, Lee KM, Kim J. Higher operating table for optimal needle-entry angle and less discomfort during spinal anesthesia. Anesth Analg. 2018;126(4):1349.
5. Cesarano FL, Piergeorge AR. The spaghetti syndrome. A new clinical entity. Crit Care Med. 1979;7(4):182–3.
6. Ofek E, Pizov R, Bitterman N. From a radial operating theatre to a self-contained operating table. Anaesthesia. 2006;61(6):548–52.
7. Bayramzadeh S, Joseph A, Allison D, Shultz J, Abernathy J, RIPCHD.OR Study Group. Using an integrative mock-up simulation approach for evidence-based evaluation of operating room design prototypes. Appl Ergon. 2018;70:288–99.
8. Hodge B, Thompson JF. Noise pollution in the operating theatre. Lancet. 1990;335(8694):891–4.
9. Fritsch MH, Chacko CE, Patterson EB. Operating room sound level hazards for patients and physicians. Otol Neurotol. 2010;31(5):715.
10. Schmid F, Goepfert MS, Kuhnt D, Eichhorn V, Diedrichs S, Reichenspurner H, et al. The wolf is crying in the operating room: patient monitor and anesthesia workstation alarming patterns during cardiac surgery. Anesth Analg. 2011;112(1):78.
11. Wiegmann DA, ElBardissi AW, Dearani JA, Daly RC, Sundt TM. Disruptions in surgical flow and their relationship to surgical errors: an exploratory investigation. Surgery. 2007;142(5):658–65.
12. Betza SM, Jurewicz KA, Neyens DM, Riggs SL, Abernathy JH, Reeves ST. Anesthesia maintenance and vigilance: examining task switching. Proceedings of the Human Factors and Ergonomics Society Annual Meeting, Sage/Los Angeles: SAGE Publications, 2016;60(1):608–612.
13. Pfeffer S, Maier T, Stricker E, Rall M, Trick M. Cognitive ergonomics and informatory load in anesthesia. Biom Eng. 2012;57(SI-1 Track-J):947–50. Available from: https://www.degruyter.com/view/j/bmte.2012.57.issue-s1-J/bmt-2012-4305/bmt-2012-4305.xml.
14. Epstein RH, Dexter F, Gratch DM, Lubarsky DA. Intraoperative handoffs among anesthesia providers increase the incidence of documentation errors for controlled drugs. Jt Comm J Qual Patient Saf. 2017;43(8):396–402.

15. Wadhera RK, Parker SH, Burkhart HM, Greason KL, Neal JR, Levenick KM, et al. Is the "sterile cockpit" concept applicable to cardiovascular surgery critical intervals or critical events? The impact of protocol-driven communication during cardiopulmonary bypass. J Thorac Cardiovasc Surg. 2010;139(2):312–9.
16. Guttman O, Lazzara E, Keebler J, Webster KL, Gisick L, Baker A. Dissecting communication barriers in healthcare: a path to enhancing communication resiliency, reliability, and patient safety. J Patient Saf. 2018; [cited 2019 Nov 15];Publish Ahead of Print. Available from: insights.ovid.com.
17. Atcherson SR, Mendel LL, Baltimore WJ, Patro C, Lee S, Pousson M, et al. The effect of conventional and transparent surgical masks on speech understanding in individuals with and without hearing loss. J Am Acad Audiol. 2017;28(1):58–67.
18. Pauchot J, Meresse T, Di Tommaso L, Grumblat A, Samain E, Obert L, et al. Le champ de tête transparent. Un moyen simple de prévention des accidents liés au changement d'installation en chirurgie plastique. Annales de Chirurgie Plastique Esthétique. 2010;55(6):587–92.
19. Hawksworth C, Asbury AJ, Millar K. Music in theatre: not so harmonious. Anaesthesia. 1997;52(1):79–83.
20. Hawksworth CRE, Sivalingam P, Asbury AJ. The effect of music on anaesthetists' psychomotor performance. Anaesthesia. 1998;53(2):195–7.

Human Factors in Military Surgery

10

Jason Nam and Matthew J. Martin

Military Surgery Overview

Modern battlefield medical and surgical care is characterized by a dangerous and rapidly changing environment, limited resources, and challenges due to the number of casualties and the severity of their injuries. After 18 years of war against violent extremist organizations, the military has constantly evolved to fight a determined foe. Military surgeons have concurrently had to adopt a mentality of developing new best clinical practices, sharing them, and learning new advanced procedures for this new way of warfare [1].

Case Study: To better understand how human factors led to a well-designed military medical care system that provides the highest possible care in severely challenging environments, here are two case studies.

Point-of-Injury and Resuscitation

Somewhere in the Middle East, on a joint combat patrol, one US soldier and one partner force soldier suffered dismounted blast and fragmentation injuries from an improvised explosive device (IED). They were transported by non-medics in the bed of a pick-up truck to a US Army forward damage control resuscitation (DCR) team staffed by a physician and combat medics within 30 minutes of injury. They were positioned in a building of opportunity, and no pre-hospital field interventions had been performed [2].

J. Nam
Department of Medicine, Womack Army Medical Center, Fort Bragg, NC, USA

M. J. Martin (✉)
Trauma and Emergency Surgery Service, Department of Surgery, Scripps Mercy Hospital, San Diego, CA, USA

T. N. Cohen et al. (eds.), *Human Factors in Surgery*,
https://doi.org/10.1007/978-3-030-53127-0_10

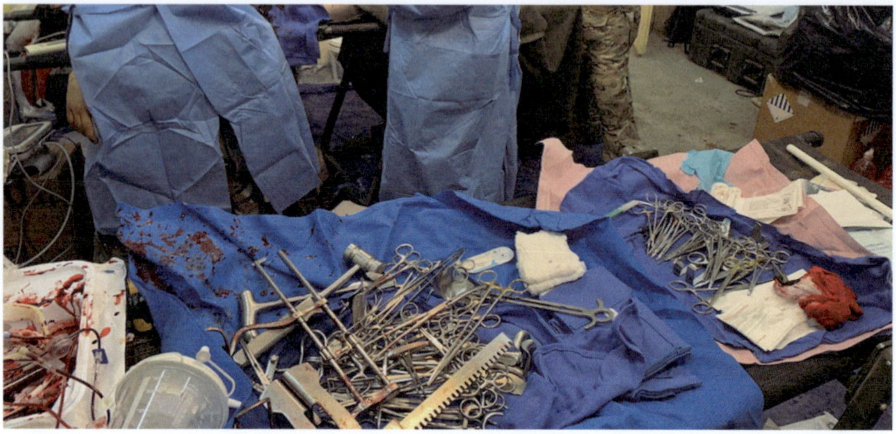

Fig. 10.1 US forward damage control surgery team operating in a building of opportunity at an austere location

On arrival, patient Alpha was hypotensive with extensive fragmentation wounds and a mangled right lower extremity with a partial amputation at the level of the mid-tibia. During resuscitation, an extended focused assessment with sonography for trauma (eFAST) was positive in the abdomen. Patient Bravo suffered a right open tibia-fibula fracture, left femur fracture, and extensive fragmentation injuries. An eFAST exam was similarly positive in the abdomen. A partner force ambulance transported both patients to a US Air Force damage control surgery (DCS) team located 45 minutes away (Fig. 10.1) [2].

Surgical Facility Care

The DCS team consisting of a single surgeon operated out of a makeshift building. Both patients arrived hypotensive and confused. A right-sided chest tube was placed in Patient Bravo for pneumothorax without any significant blood output. At this time, it was recognized that both patients required immediate surgery with only one surgeon and operating room available. The decision was made by the surgeon to place resuscitative endovascular balloon occlusion of aorta (REBOA) catheters in both patients [2].

An ER physician placed one of the REBOA catheters. Patient Bravo was taken to the OR. Exploratory laparotomy was performed with extensive lysis of adhesions, mesenteric hemorrhage control, multiple enterotomy repairs, ascending colon resection, and abdominal washout and packing. Total OR time was approximately 1.5 hours. While awaiting surgery, the resuscitation team maintained Patient Alpha's SBP with transfusion of four units of Low O-titer Whole Blood (LTOWB). He underwent exploratory laparotomy with mesenteric bleeding control, ileocecectomy, and multiple small bowel resections [2].

Postoperatively, both patients maintained hemodynamic stability and were noted to be making urine. Patient Alpha was the partner force (host nation) soldier. He survived the 4-hour transport to the next level of care. We were unable to get any outcomes from the local partner forces due to active fighting and significant distance between sites. Patient Bravo was the US soldier. He survived successive transfers of care to include follow-on surgeries at a role III hospital. Within 48 hours of injury, Patient Bravo had consecutive critical care air transport transfers to Germany and then onto Walter Reed National Medical Center for definitive surgery. The cases and care of both patients were reviewed at all echelons throughout this continuum and discussed on a weekly system-wide video conference call that included the relevant providers involved in these cases from the point-of-injury through to the hospital in the United States.

Analysis

There were extensive rehearsals and preparation prior to arrival. Because of the austere nature of their work, both DCR and DCS teams did extensive field training and practice doing medicine in resource-limited areas. The DCR and DCS teams completed rehearsals together, so that patient care and transfer would be seamless. Both patients had casualty care cards filled out with vital sign trends and interventions performed. The DCR physician called the DCS surgeon to give a "doc-to-doc" hand out prior to patient transfer. Though the REBOA procedure is commonly reserved for surgeons, the DCS surgeon had done extensive training with the ER provider in case there are more patients requiring a REBOA catheter. All of the critical aspects of care in this patient, including resuscitation, REBOA, initial evaluation, and surgical interventions, were covered in an up-to-date set of clinical practice guidelines (CPGs) for combat casualty care developed by the Joint Trauma System (JTS).

Patient Alpha was a partner force soldier and was ultimately "lost to follow-up." This is a fairly common occurrence in the deployed setting when our partners have their own respective healthcare systems that vary widely in capabilities, capacity, and quality. With no feedback, there is little room for process improvement. Patient Bravo's journey to the United States highlights multiple key areas where the US military medical system functioned well: communication between successive echelons of medical care, seamless patient handoffs and tracking across three continents, and a well-led process honed by years of war. However, it is critical to note that many of these systems and processes were not in existence at the beginning of combat operations in the Middle East, but instead had to be developed and adopted based on real-time experience and lessons learned from deployed providers and medical/surgical units.

How Military Surgeons Use Human Factor Principles

The Global War on Terrorism (GWOT) has been ongoing for 18 years (at the time of this writing) across a wide geographic territory, which includes Asia, Africa, Europe, and the Middle East. To support such disparate combat operations, military surgeons have been placed in a variety of remote locations and austere settings. Furthermore, enemies have evolved their combat tactics and procedures to defeat US and coalition forces.

The ubiquitous improvised explosive device (IED) has evolved as coalition forces developed countermeasures. In doing so, combat wounds and injuries have become increasingly complex and devastating. Surgeons have had to share best practices and also continuously adopt new and evolving practices as the battlefield has changed. Lastly, battlefield commanders have increasingly pushed military surgeons further forward, requiring surgeons to be able to transfer patients and communicate with other surgeons at different echelons usually several time zones away. All of these factors make the establishment and implementation of an effective, reliable, and well-ordered system of care extremely difficult. Arguably, of most importance from a human factors design standpoint is the superimposed challenge of constantly changing and rotating personnel, with physicians and other key personnel being replaced as frequently as every 3–6 months. This resulted in noticeable declines in the quality of care immediately following handoffs to a new and inexperienced team and early individualized efforts to preserve and pass on critical information and lessons learned (Table 10.1).

With wars being waged in Afghanistan and Iraq, in 2004, the US Assistant Secretary of Defense (ASD), Health Affairs (HA), ordered all respective military services to work together to establish a single trauma registry and deployed trauma system. The ASD (HA) Policy Memorandum 04-03, Coordination of Policy to Establish a Joint Theater Trauma Registry was a mandate for all services to collect and aggregate combat casualty care epidemiology, treatments, and outcomes [3, 4]. This was essential to understanding the challenges, successes, and failures that

Table 10.1 Example of a unit-specific document used to pass on key lessons to incoming personnel—top 10 list of lessons from the 28th Combat Support Hospital, Baghdad, Iraq in 2008

Top ten combat trauma lessons
1. Patients die in the emergency room, and
2. Patients die in the CT scanner
3. Therefore, a hypotensive trauma patient belongs in the operating room ASAP
4. Most blown up or shot patients need blood products, not crystalloids. Avoid trying "hypotensive resuscitation"; it is for civilian trauma.
5. For mangled extremities and amputations, one code red (which allows immediate blood availability) per extremity started as soon as they arrive.
6. Patients in extremis will code during rapid sequence intubation, be prepared, and intubate these patients in the OR (not the ER) whenever possible.
7. This hospital can go from empty to full in a matter of hours; don't be lulled by the slow periods.
8. The name of the game here is not continuity of care, it is throughput. If the ICU or wards are full, you are mission incapable.
9. MASCALs live or die by proper triage and prioritization—starting at the door and including which X-rays to get, labs, and disposition.
10. No Personal Projects!!! They clog the system, waste resources, and anger others.

Reprinted with permission from: Martin et al. [1]

military medicine faced in providing effective and timely care for combat casualties and to implement rapid solutions to pressing problems/challenges identified in real-time. In order to help manage this registry, the Joint Trauma System (JTS) was created to build and manage the Department of Defense (DoD) Trauma Registry (DODTR). This is a critical resource to validate and analyze collected data, provide data-driven system-wide quality/process improvement efforts (Fig. 10.2), and act as an advisory resource to combatant commanders on combat trauma-related topics [3, 4]. By 2016, the Office of the Under Secretary of Defense for Personnel and Readiness recommended the DoD "establish the JTS, in its role as the DoD Trauma System as the lead agency for trauma in DoD with authority to establish and assure best practice trauma care guidelines to the Director of the Defense Health Agency, the Services, and the Combatant Commanders" [3].

Establishment of the JTS is arguably the most important human factors event that occurred in modern battlefield medical care for the US military. This ensured a central agent that assumed responsibility for the conduct and quality of forward trauma care. One of the earliest initiatives of the newly formed JTS was to establish the weekly combat casualty care video teleconference call series. This call is used to discuss the care of casualties at all deployed US medical treatment facilities and to provide feedback from the various echelons along the chain of care. The teleconference is open to all relevant military and civilian providers to discuss individual patient care issues, local/regional issues, and system-wide processes that need to be

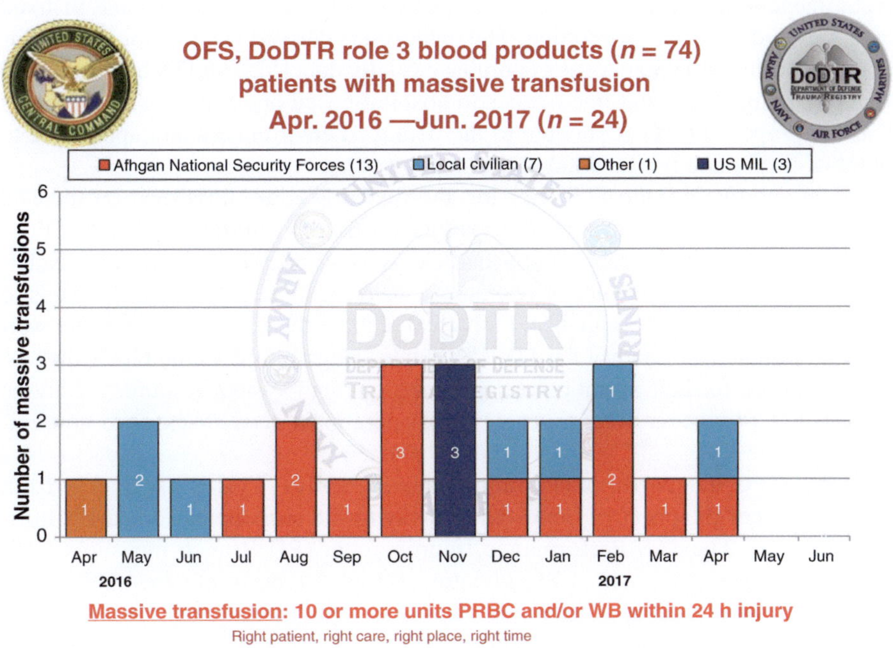

Fig. 10.2 Example slide from a Joint Trauma System standard report characterizing massive transfusion trends over time in 2017

improved and adjusted. This is also used as a means to track patients as they progress through the casualty evacuation chain. The JTS Combat Casualty Care conference has been held weekly since 2005 and has expanded in scope to be open to all members of our trauma system team [5]. This provides near real-time feedback on trauma care outcomes and recent patients. The conference also highlights the critical work military surgeons perform in assessing and improving outcomes. This conference serves as a model for communication and inclusion, shared awareness, and validation of the contributions of all members to improve trauma and combat casualty care outcomes [5, 6].

Clinical Practice Guidelines (CPGs) are the backbone of the system-wide JTS Performance Improvement (PI) program. Health data abstracted from patient records and after-action reports are analyzed and distilled into globally relevant CPGs to remove medical practice variations and prevent needless deaths. These are updated frequently to establish best practices. It allows for greater uniformity of practices across military surgeons doing surgery in a variety of locations and echelons of care [6]. The CPGs are developed by clinical Subject Matter Experts (SME) in response to needs identified in the particular area of operations. The proposed topic usually identifies a perceived gap in care and would drive changes in performance [7]. The JTS CPGs are evidenced-based as best as possible, although the degree and quality of evidentiary support varies widely based on the topic and the available relevant literature. Although they frequently parallel guidelines for civilian trauma care, there are often significant differences in the approach or recommendations because much of combat casualty care occurs outside of fixed hospitals and in an austere setting. The evidence is derived from the published literature or internal JTS analysis of combat casualty data [5]. The JTS has a working group ranging from front line medics to hospital-based physicians, which ensures that the proposed CPG is suitable to the deployed environment and applicable to point-of-injury and pre-hospital phases of care [7].

Upon approval by the JTS Director, the final CPGs are published on the JTS website and are publicly available (https://jts.amedd.army.mil/index.cfm/PI_CPGs/cpgs). The JTS sends recently published CPGs to all relevant medical and leadership personnel in that theater of operations, who then share it with their teams to ensure awareness and compliance. Individual units or theater commanders are welcome to utilize or to modify the JTS CPGs into geographic-specific CPGs that are better tailored to their specific area of operations and system resources. Routine updates to CPGs occur every 5 years, as the operational need arises, or as new evidence surfaces [8].

Every CPG has performance improvement metrics. This is applicable from the medic near the point of injury all the way to the surgeon at a fixed US military hospital. The JTS Performance Improvement (PI) Branch measures CPG adherence through the use of PI indicators, which are built into each CPG plan. Each CPG is assigned up to four core measures—quality indicators [8]. Tracking the core measures exposes deficiencies that are addressed by providing education, material solutions, or improving processes. The JTS also provides solutions as "good," "better," and "best," so that providers in resource-limited settings can approach clinical problems in a stepwise fashion.

Unfortunately, there still remains a significant deviation in the adherence to CPGs. A recent review of US military surgical practices in Operation Inherent Resolve (Iraq-Syria) found significant variability in surgical adherence to these CPGs despite widespread emphasis on their importance from the medical leadership [9]. There have also been ongoing problems with ensuring that all providers deploying to one of the current combat theaters are aware of the existence of CPGs, know how to access them, and are familiar with their scope and content. This represents an ongoing human factor challenge that the JTS and military medicine continue to struggle with, and that is made more challenging by the frequent turnover of personnel both within the military services and in staffing of the forward military treatment facilities.

However, one major success story involving CPGs is the use of whole blood (WB) transfusion. Initially, at the onset of the wars in Iraq and Afghanistan, the US military medical teams were using component therapy comprising individual packed red blood cells, plasma, and platelet products. With subsequent publication of the Pragmatic, Randomized Optimal Platelet and Plasma Ratios (PROPPR) Trial, it was found that in patients with severe trauma and major bleeding, early administration of plasma, platelets, and red blood cells in a 1:1:1 ratio vs 1:1:2 ratio did not result in significant differences in mortality at 24 hours or 30 days [10]. However, more patients in the 1:1:1 group achieved hemostasis, and fewer experienced death due to exsanguination at 24 hours [10]. Such scientific evidence has forced the US military to evolve to the point that now WB is readily available for transfusion among most military aid stations, deployed surgical teams, and larger combat support hospitals [11]. WB transfusion is a standard of practice that has been demonstrated to result in superior outcomes among combat casualties and that has particular benefits in the austere setting due to its ease of use compared to individual component blood products [11]. Even Special Operations Forces (SOF) medics will now go on missions with several units of Low O-titer WB (LTOWB).

The sporadic nature of trauma in a deployed setting and the need to frequently draw providers from outside the organic surgical team necessitate the need for frequent rehearsals. This is particularly true for mass casualty events (MASCAL), which are inherently chaotic and challenging in an already chaotic "fog of war" situation. In such incidents, military surgical team members will have defined responsibilities to include triage, DCR, and initiating a walking blood bank. Especially since these teams have members with a wide range of experience and training, MASCAL rehearsals are often the first things a team will accomplish upon arriving at a deployed setting [12]. The most critical factors to the recognized success of forward military units in dealing with multiple MASCAL situations have been the system-wide emphasis on frequent and realistic MASCAL preparation and training (Fig. 10.3), the requirement for units to have a well-developed written MASCAL plan, and the capture of key lessons learned and best practices [13].

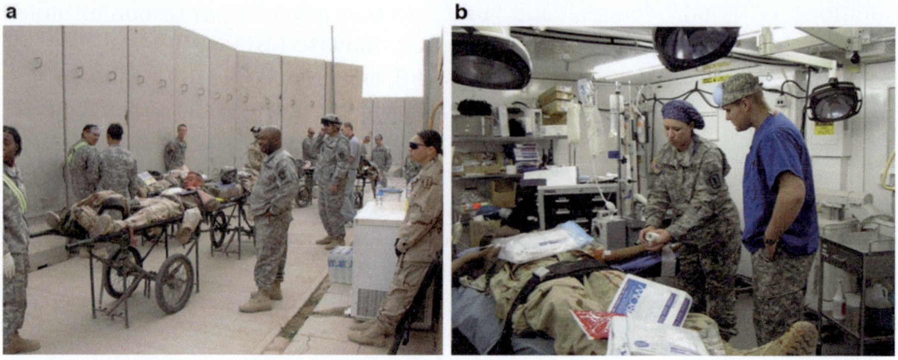

Fig. 10.3 Mass casualty exercise being performed at a Combat Support Hospital in Iraq as part of the turnover process to a new medical team, emphasizing (**a**) realistic scenarios with live patients and (**b**) continuing the exercise through to the operating room and subsequent preparation for transfer

As the US military continues to push surgeons into forward remote areas, the surgeon is often task-saturated, especially in a situation such as MASCAL. Teaching of advanced procedures to non-surgeon providers such as REBOA is critical and physician-extending. There are now examples of US military non-surgeons placing a REBOA as a lifesaving adjunct to stabilize a severely injured casualty while awaiting surgery [14]. And there are programs in place with Special Forces units to train their advanced combat paramedics to first learn how to place a REBOA catheter and how to do so on an aerial evacuation platform [15, 16]. Both examples highlight the importance of realistic and effective training paradigms, communication, and rehearsals.

As with our Patients Alpha and Bravo, since military surgeons often require transfer of patients to higher levels of command, communication is critically important. In the initial years of the current combat experience, there were significant challenges to communicating critical medical information from one location to the next along the echelon of care, leading to fragmentation and medical errors or major lapses. Individual workarounds such as documenting directly on patient dressings or sending handwritten notes were common, but were sporadic and non-standardized (Fig. 10.4). The military has since adopted standardized and more universal approaches to documentation and medical records, including the use of a tactical combat casualty care (TCCC) card (Fig. 10.4b), a standardized Joint Theater Trauma Registry (JTTR) chart, and a universal web-based electronic medical record (EMR) system [7]. The TCCC card is more often completed by the medic or buddy at point-of-injury. It allows the start of medical documentation of injuries, vitals, physical exam, medications administered, and interventions performed. By the time the patient has been seen by a provider in a Role II setting, a physician or surgeon has begun to chart on the JTTR paper chart and data is then entered into the EMR [7].

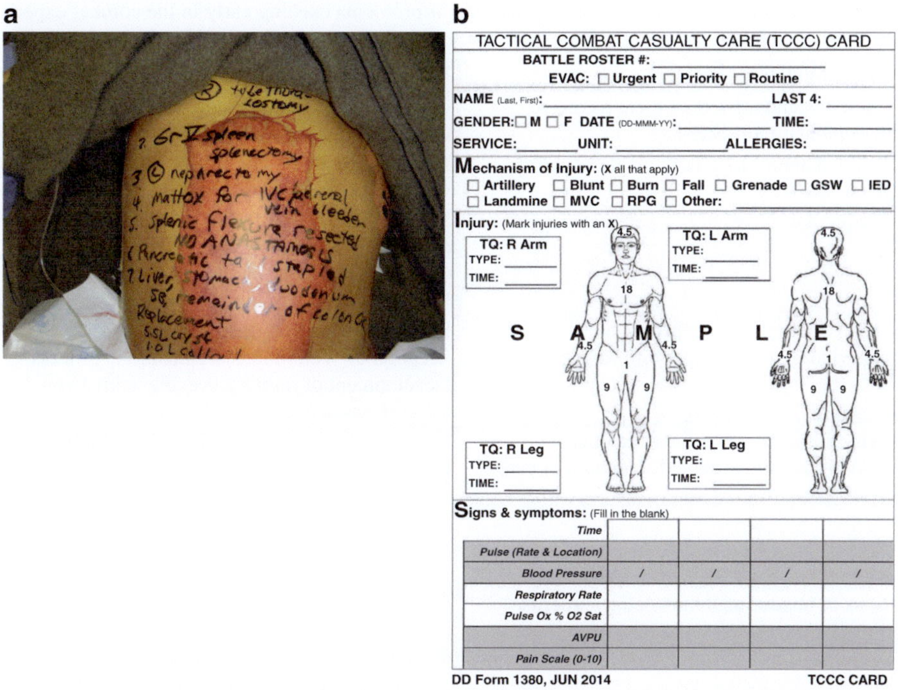

Fig. 10.4 (**a**) Handwritten documentation on the abdominal dressing of a patient transferred between facilities and (**b**) tactical combat casualty care card subsequently introduced to facilitate and standardize documentation

Lessons Learned/Personal Pearls

- The more austere, chaotic, and resource limited the environment, the greater the need for a human factors approach to ensure consistent, safe, and high-quality care.
- Individual and "personality driven" processes of care can be effective in the short term, but long-term solutions require embedded and system-wide processes.
- Robust data collection and real-time analysis are the cornerstones of trauma quality improvement—you are only ever as good as your data.
- Periods of key personnel turnover/handoffs are particularly vulnerable to declines in the quality of care and require focused attention and processes to avoid preventable morbidity and mortality.
- The US military achieved remarkable improvements in combat casualty care by centralizing responsibility and accountability for battlefield trauma care in one agency, the Joint Trauma System, and implementing numerous "failsafe" processes/programs (Table 10.2)

Table 10.2 Sample of major initial limitations or problems existing early in the combat experience and the human factors programs or interventions that were implemented to address them

Initial limitations/problems	Intervention or programs implemented
Lack of standardized medical record or documentation process	Creation of templated medical record form CPG on medical documentation
Limited ability to communicate between locations	Introduction of low bandwidth EMRs and web-based medical records systems
Frequent turnover of key personnel/expertise	Standardized hand-off process during personnel changes Creation of "living" documents capturing key lessons
Inconsistent trauma expertise and level of experience among deploying surgeons	Standardized pre-deployment training Creation of "continuous certification" process Development of military-specific animal and cadaver-based courses
Wide variations in patient care and deviations from accepted standards of care	Creation of evidence-based CPGs on high priority topics Standardized pre-deployment CPG familiarization training Weekly JTS teleconference and patient care review
Loss of institutional knowledge/expertise	Creation of multiple textbooks to capture and pass on critical knowledge and lessons to new deployers Partnering with civilian trauma organizations to enhance mentoring and education of military surgeons
No organized trauma system in place	Establishment of Joint Trauma System
No universal and standardized data collection	Establishment of Department of Defense Trauma Registry
Inability to address system-wide issues/problems	Weekly JTS teleconference and patient care review Deployment of dedicated JTS personnel to theater Routine data review and process improvement filters
No local or regional authority in the combat theater with oversight and ownership of combat casualty care	Creation of a Theater Trauma Director in each major theater of operations, filled by an experienced trauma surgeon
Lack of coordination/communication between pre-hospital, en-route, and in-hospital personnel	Elevation of JTS to position of responsibility/authority Coordination between DCOTs responsible for pre-hospital, en-route, and in-hospital combat casualty care

CPG clinical practice guideline, *JTS* Joint Trauma System, *DCOTs* Defense Committees on Trauma

References

1. Martin M, Beekley A, Eckert M. Front line surgery: a practical approach. 2nd ed. New York: Springer; 2017. xxii, 533pp
2. Manley J, Le AT, Nam JJ. A case report of simultaneous hypotensive patients managed with concurrent REBOA in a single-surgeon, austere combat casualty environment. J Endovasc Resusc Trauma Manag. 2018;2(2):77–80.
3. System JT. Department of Defense Instruction 6040.47: Department of Defense; 2016. Updated 28 Sept 2016. Available from: https://jts.amedd.army.mil/assets/docs/policies/JTS-DoDI-604047.pdf.
4. Holcomb JB, Stansbury LG, Champion HR, Wade C, Bellamy RF. Understanding combat casualty care statistics. J Trauma. 2006;60(2):397–401.
5. Eastridge BJ, Wade CE, Spott MA, Costanzo G, Dunne J, Flaherty S, et al. Utilizing a trauma systems approach to benchmark and improve combat casualty care. J Trauma. 2010;69(Suppl 1):S5–9.
6. Butler FK Jr, Blackbourne LH. Battlefield trauma care then and now: a decade of Tactical Combat Casualty Care. J Trauma Acute Care Surg. 2012;73(6 Suppl 5):S395–402.
7. Eastridge BJ, Costanzo G, Jenkins D, Spott MA, Wade C, Greydanus D, et al. Impact of joint theater trauma system initiatives on battlefield injury outcomes. Am J Surg. 2009;198(6):852–7.
8. Spott MA, Burelison DR, Kurkowski CR, Stockinger ZT. JTS CPG development process. Mil Med. 2018;183(suppl_2):12–4.
9. Plackett TP, Cherry DC, Delk G, Satterly S, Theler J, McVay D, et al. Clinical practice guideline adherence during Operation Inherent Resolve. J Trauma Acute Care Surg. 2017;83(1 Suppl 1):S66–s70.
10. Holcomb JB, Tilley BC, Baraniuk S, Fox EE, Wade CE, Podbielski JM, et al. Transfusion of plasma, platelets, and red blood cells in a 1:1:1 vs a 1:1:2 ratio and mortality in patients with severe trauma: the PROPPR randomized clinical trial. JAMA. 2015;313(5):471–82.
11. Vanderspurt CK, Spinella PC, Cap AP, Hill R, Matthews SA, Corley JB, et al. The use of whole blood in US military operations in Iraq, Syria, and Afghanistan since the introduction of low-titer type O whole blood: feasibility, acceptability, challenges. Transfusion. 2019;59(3):965–70.
12. Benavides JM, Benavides LC, Hale DF, Lundy JB. The golden hour offset surgical treatment team operational concept: experience of the 102nd forward surgical team in Operation Freedom's Sentinel 2015–2016. J Spec Oper Med. 2017;17(3):46–50.
13. Kuckelman J, Derickson M, Long WB, Martin MJ. MASCAL management from Baghdad to Boston: top ten lessons learned from modern military and civilian MASCAL events. Curr Trauma Rep. 2018;4:138–48.
14. Lyon RF, Northern DM. REBOA by a non-surgeon as an adjunct during MASCAL. Am J Emerg Med. 2018;36(6):1121.e5–6.
15. Redman TT, Ross EM. A novel expeditionary perfused cadaver model for trauma training in the out-of-hospital setting. J Emerg Med. 2018;55(3):383–9.
16. Ross EM, Redman TT. Feasibility and proposed training pathway for austere application of resuscitative balloon occlusion of the aorta. J Spec Oper Med. 2018;18(1):37–43.

Enhancing Safety and Efficiency in Robotic Surgery

11

Monica Jain, Kate Cohen, and Daniel Shouhed

What Is Robotic Surgery?

Robotic surgery, or robot-assisted surgery, is a type of minimally invasive procedure performed with a camera and small keyhole incisions through which instruments are inserted. In contrast to laparoscopic surgery, a surgeon performing robotic surgery sits comfortably at a console away from the patient, at which they are able to: 1) look through a screen that provides improved visualization via 3-dimensional optics, 2) control the movements of up to four robotic arms, and 3) enjoy increased manipulation and articulation of instruments through the use of joysticks. Robotic surgery offers improved visualization, ergonomics, precision, and autonomy compared to conventional laparoscopic surgery.

Case Study

Below are two case studies that may help characterize how human factors can facilitate better system design within robotic surgery to provide the best possible care, or alternatively, prevent catastrophe.

When Things Go Wrong

A young male is being prepped and draped in the operating room in preparation for a robotic right inguinal hernia repair with mesh. The attending surgeon has performed 50 robotic cases and is planning to take his surgical resident through the case. He is unaware that both the resident and scrub technician are participating in

M. Jain · K. Cohen · D. Shouhed (✉)
Department of Surgery, Cedars-Sinai Medical Center, Los Angeles, CA, USA
e-mail: daniel.shouhed@cshs.org

T. N. Cohen et al. (eds.), *Human Factors in Surgery*,
https://doi.org/10.1007/978-3-030-53127-0_11

their first robotic case. The circulating nurse attempts to dock the robot but struggles due to the small size of the room and collisions with the overhead lights. She then trips over the electric cords, which causes an unrecoverable fault, requiring the robotic system to be reset. After a more than 20-minute delay, the arms are docked. One of the instruments typically used for this procedure has expired and the nurse must go to a different floor to obtain another one. The robot is finally docked with the appropriate instruments, enabling the attending and resident to sit at the console. When asked to "burp back" one of the robotic trocars, the nurse inadvertently removes the entire trocar, requiring the attending to scrub back in to re-insert the trocar. The resident is struggling to perform basic tasks despite the attending's efforts to train him. The attending is also training the scrub technician via verbal instruction on how to perform basic tasks, such as instrument exchanges and camera cleaning. The scrub technician then removes the instrument from the incorrect arm, which was holding onto a vessel, leading to significant bleeding. The bleeding is controlled, however, the case requires an additional 90 minutes to complete. After removing all of the trocars and closing the incisions, the nurse informs the attending that the needle count is incorrect. The abdomen is re-explored and the needle is found, adding additional time to the case.

Analysis: The case above demonstrates a cascade of errors and disruptions in the flow of an operation that ultimately led to an adverse event and a near miss. Although the attending surgeon was nearly past his learning curve, the other members of the team, including the surgical resident, scrub technician, and circulating nurse, were not. Inefficient docking of the robot caused the initial delay, leading to frustration and a break in the flow of the operation, a key contributor to subsequent flow disruptions and errors. The attending surgeon could have prevented some of the issues that occurred by using a more methodical preoperative approach. He might have communicated ahead of time what instruments he needed, or might have demonstrated how to dock the robot before scrubbing out. Better team communication or more extensive training may have prevented the inadvertent removal of the instrument that led to bleeding. Tasks that are typically easy to perform were difficult for the team members, requiring more focus on the part of the novice individuals to perform basic tasks and requiring the attending to expend significant attention on training others. These distractions led to operative delays and an inaccurately performed needle count, which led to a near miss event.

When a System Functions Well

You are scheduled to perform a robotic gastric bypass, an operation that involves extensive operative steps, instrument exchanges, and technical expertise. Before the start of the case, you performed a team huddle, alerting the anesthesiologist to the need for a sizing tube and suggested how much fluid to give during the case. You also inform the circulating nurse and the scrub technician what instruments, sutures, and other equipment you will need during the case. Prior to scrubbing the case, you move all barriers that may be in the way of the robot when it is to be docked, such as overhead lights, towers, and electrical cords. In addition to a scrub technician, you have a physician assistant (PA) who has done countless robotic cases with you, particularly robotic gastric bypasses. You place your ports and dock the robot and the robotic arms within 3 minutes. All instruments are connected and you scrub out to get on the console with your senior resident, who has been practicing on the robotic simulator and has watched several videos pertinent to the technical details of the case. As you progress through the case, you inform the scrub technician and PA in advance what instruments will need to be exchanged and what sutures will need to be placed so they have time to prepare. As the PA removes one instrument, the scrub replaces it with another, in sync with one another, to seamlessly maintain the perfect flow of the operation. The attending surgeon repeats each request, which the PA then repeats back. At one point during the case, you notice limited intra-abdominal space to work and the PA immediately resolves the problem after realizing he had forgotten to place the 8-mm reducer into the 12-mm robotic trocar. You encounter bleeding from a short gastric vessel, which is quickly controlled as you have suction connected, a sponge already placed in the abdomen, and a clip applier in the room ready to be opened. The case concludes in 2 hours and the patient has an uneventful recovery.

Analysis: The case above demonstrates how a case runs smoothly when the right preparations, training, and communication have been employed. Preoperative planning is crucial, which, in the scenario above, led to a timely, inconsequential recovery during the bleeding event. Communication was excellent during the case and requests were recited back to ensure the proper exchange of instruments, efficient insertion of sutures, and speedy replacement of instruments. Despite minor complications and interruptions, such as bleeding and loss of insufflation, the procedure progressed without incident, as each participant knew their role and executed each task deliberately, safely, and effectively.

How Can We Improve the Safety and Efficiency of Robotic Surgery Using Human Factors Principles?

Situation Awareness and Training

As our knowledge and understanding of medicine continues to evolve, so does the technology that enables physicians to provide medical treatment and surgical care. Over the past 20 years, the field of surgery has reached a new frontier - robotic surgery has penetrated nearly every specialty of surgery. The da Vinci robot provides a platform that enables surgeons to perform an operation while sitting comfortably with a console, viewing the operation through a 3-dimensional screen, and controlling four articulating arms through the use of two joysticks. Most would argue that robotic surgery, as compared to conventional laparoscopic surgery, provides superior ergonomics, better visualization, greater precision, and more autonomy.

Greater complexities, opportunities for inefficiencies, and potential safety hazards accompany these technologic advancements and expansion into new surgical tools and equipment. In the traditional surgical setting, surgical team members are centered around the patient and the operating room table. Even in complex cases when there are additions to the surgical team, such as endovascular technicians or perfusionists, surgical team members are in close proximity to and are able to interact with one another constantly. The surgeon relies on her assistant(s) for visualization, retraction, dissection, and other critical portions of the operation. In addition, the surgeon is in constant communication with the surgical technician for instrument management. The majority of interactions occur face-to-face, although non-verbal interactions make up a significant portion of all communication around the operating room table.

Robotic surgery changes the spatial configuration of the operating room. The surgeon is now seated at the robotic console, removed from the patient and the majority of the surgical team. He relies on the first assistant and surgical technician to provide direct assistance at the bedside. The surgeon views the operation through a set of lenses with his entire visual field focused solely on the telescopic operative field. Unless the surgeon removes his head from within the console, he has no view of what is happening in the surrounding environment. Thus, the surgeon becomes more dependent on his other senses, such as hearing, and auditory signals from the robotic system and anesthesia machine have much greater bearing. Finally, as face-to-face interactions are not feasible, verbal communication from the anesthesiologist and the staff are critically important during robotic surgery.

Situation awareness is an essential non-technical skill, defined as "the perception of elements in the environment, comprehension of their meaning, and the projection of their status in the near future" [2, 3]. Certain disciplines demand heightened situation awareness due to an expanded operating room staff (e.g. cardiac surgery and the addition of a perfusionist); however, in these cases, all of the surgical team members are still at the operative field and within reach [2]. In robotic surgery, the physical separation of the surgeon at the console makes situation awareness an especially critical behavioral skill. Poor situation awareness may be detrimental to the quality of intraoperative decision-making [3].

It would be deceptive to assert that the surgeon alone is responsible for being cognizant of the operating room environment. Team situation awareness depends on the shared goal of responsibility for the wider operating room between the surgeon, the anesthesiologist, and the staff. The surgeon must rely partly on the other members of the operating room team to transmit information about the status of the patient since she cannot see the patient [3]. In this regard, non-verbal communication amongst the staff facilitates monitoring of the operating room and bolsters team situation awareness [3]. Importantly, excellent team situation awareness can act as a safeguard to degraded surgeon situation awareness.

Traditional laparoscopy and robotic surgery share the need for deliberate practice dedicated to the attainment of discrete technical goals in a non-clinical environment in order to develop long-term expertise [4]. However, to date, there is no established and validated comprehensive, standardized curriculum for robotic surgery [4]. Furthermore, the unique complexities and configurations of robotic surgery demand new technical and non-technical skills that call for innovation in training programs beyond what currently exists. Simulation alone cannot fully communicate the additional skills needed in robotic surgery, which must be learned through both training and experience [4–6]. It is crucial that training also takes place in the clinical setting so that trainees may experience first-hand typical issues during robotic surgery and strengthen their situation awareness.

Due to the difficulties of conducting mentored intraoperative teaching in robotic surgery, training approaches have relied upon techniques such as needs assessments to develop proficiency-based curricula based on deconstructed skills, ex post facto flow disruption analyses, and simulation [4, 5]. Even these methods have drawbacks, such as the high cost of the supplies used for simulated training (e.g. sutures and robotic instruments). Furthermore, there are few standard metrics for measuring progress in proficiency [4].

Experienced surgeons progressively develop situation awareness and respond better to visual cues. For example, greater familiarity with the robot leads to fewer robotic arm collisions and shorter operative time [3]. The same is true of experienced operating room staff and bedside assistants. A properly trained bedside assistant is crucial in robotic surgery due to the spatial separation of the surgeon from the operating room table while on the console. Assistant-made errors may lead to severe consequences, including higher rates of complications, retained foreign items, and conversion to open surgery, in addition to inefficiency in operative time and increased lengths of stay. Going forward, there may be a need for earlier and more formal training programs specifically geared towards bedside assistants in robotic surgery [7].

Operating Room Turnover

The time required to clean and prepare an operating room between two surgical cases is commonly referred to as turnover time (TOT). The addition of a robot in the operating room requires better communication and coordination among team members during turnover. It also requires more time to clean and prepare an additional tool with separate instruments and unique needs [8]. Unsurprisingly, research has found that turnover time for cases involving robotic surgery may be longer and more variable than those that do not utilize this technology [9]. Lowering robotic TOT has significant implications for the hospital as a whole because it can lead to improved patient and staff satisfaction as well as economic benefits.

Several approaches to reduce robotic TOT have been proposed and tested in the literature, including the introduction of process improvement methodologies like Lean and Six Sigma, workflow assessment, and redesign (e.g., applying parallel processing practices) [10]. Souders et al. applied concepts from motor racing pit stops, such as role definition, task allocation, briefings, and task sequencing, to improve robotic TOT. This method was successful in reducing turnover time from

99.2 to 53.2 minutes when measured 3 months after intervention [9]. Rebuck et al. aimed to reduce time and costs associated with robot-assisted laparoscopic radical prostatectomies via the implementation of parallel processing, the introduction of a dedicated anesthesia team to assist with setup of the robot, and removal of unused disposable equipment. These researchers were successful in reducing TOT from 43.0 to 30.9 minutes [11]. Price et al. formed a working group to review current robotic TOT practices and developed solutions for their robotic surgery program. This group reduced their robotic TOT from 59 to 49 minutes by implementing peri-operative patient care technicians and robotic staff members to support task overlap during turnover, in addition to standardizing practices of opening supplies [12]. Finally, Cohen et al. used a human factors approach to unveil the *perceived* versus *actual* barriers to efficient robotic TOT. They found that the average robotic TOT across observed cases was 72 minutes. Cleaning was the largest contributor, followed by instrument setup and patient retrieval from the pre-operative area. Survey data measuring *perceptions* of robotic TOT length and practices proved inaccurate when it came to estimating robotic TOT and predicting factors that influence TOT. The authors were also able to gain insight into individual perceptions associated with turnover and why certain behaviors occurred [13].

A multidisciplinary systems approach targeting all levels of the operating room and the hospital is required to create a cultural change amongst surgeons and staff about how robotic surgery turnovers should be addressed.

Workflow Disruptions and Team Dynamics

Flow disruptions (FDs) are deviations from the natural progression of an operation [14]. Evaluations of FDs can diagnose weaknesses in teamwork, communication, training, and other systemic factors, which can impact safety and efficiency in surgery [14, 15]. Given that robotic surgery has fundamentally changed the delivery of surgical care, the nature and frequency of FDs and the approaches to addressing them have also changed significantly. FDs occur often in robotic operations, with several studies tallying 25 to nearly 50 FDs per case [15, 16]. FD frequency is significantly greater in robotic cases than in non-robotic cases, reflecting the complex nature of robotic surgery [17]. An increased number of FDs correlates with longer operative duration; however, the precise impact of each FD is variable based on the FD type and its effect on the progression of the operation [5, 15, 16].

Most frequently, FDs in robotic surgery involve issues with coordination, communication, equipment, and training [5, 14, 15]. Further evaluation of the nature of these FDs demonstrates distinct concerns related to robotic surgery.

A major category of avoidable FDs unique to robotic surgery involved technology-related challenges. Robot docking is a process especially fraught with potential FDs due to the need for synchrony amongst the surgical team members to set up the robot for the main portion of the operation [5, 14–16]. Surgeons and the surgical team may use several different models of robotics in their regular surgical practice, further complicating the process, and changes to standard operating procedure with each successive robot model may reset the learning curve.

The altered operating room setup in robotic surgery also has significant implications for team dynamics. There may be a breakdown in the usual interactions between the surgeon and the surgical team due to the team's difficulty in anticipating the surgeon's actions when she is removed from the patient, as well as due to the lack of non-verbal communication. Multiple studies have demonstrated a significant increase in the number of communication acts during robotic surgery, as compared to that during laparoscopic surgery, due to the need for clarification or explicit feedback of various requests [1, 15]. In one study, a sub-classification of communication FDs, "repeat information," or when the surgeon has to repeat a request, accounted for approximately 60% of all communication disruptions [15]. Specifically, it was frequently observed that the surgeon had to remove her head from the console to repeat verbal commands, thereby prolonging the procedure. Although there have been attempts to address these communication issues with the installation of microphones and speakers within the robotic system, this solution is problematic as well. For example, the surgeon and the surgical team members may have difficulty hearing or understanding each other, or the surgeon may misinterpret communications meant for other members of the surgical team, leading to confusion and frustration.

Human factors interventions to decrease FDs in robotic surgery target the entire organization. Robotic surgery is a complex sociotechnical system that involves numerous stakeholders within and outside of the operating room. Team training is of the utmost importance as it allows a surgeon and their team to become familiar with the equipment, its arrangement, the necessary steps of an operation, and other technology-related concerns [3, 5, 14–16, 18–20]. Uniform deployment of team training interventions would significantly reduce coordination, equipment, and training FDs. In addition, team familiarity decreases each individual's cognitive load, resulting in fewer errors and improved efficiency [18, 20].

Communication and coordination are also improved in the setting of an experienced surgical team that is familiar with each other [1, 3, 5, 18, 20]. Most importantly, team training facilitates more effective verbal and non-verbal interaction, reduces ambiguity, and enhances safety [3, 14, 18]. To overcome challenges in communication in robotic surgery, numerous studies have emphasized the importance of "readback," in which surgical team members repeat back requests or confirm task completion in a standardized manner [1, 3, 18, 20]. This allows the surgical team to overcome the separation between the surgeon and the other team members, as well as the lack of non-verbal communication. Using explicit communication to interact with specific surgical team members is also important in reducing disruptions in the operating room [3, 18, 20]. Some surgeons have implemented new techniques that employ the robot itself to facilitate communication. For example, the surgeon could use centering/zooming with the camera and/or use the surgical instruments themselves to indicate areas of interest or issues on the camera [3, 20]. These are visible on the surgeon's console and on the screens throughout the operating room for all surgical team members to view. Such a technique enhances verbal and non-verbal interaction between team members and decreases communication-related errors [3, 20]. It also mandates that all surgical team members focus their attention on the operative case, minimizing distractions and extraneous conversations.

Finally, experience in real-life situations is an important adjunct to traditional surgical education and simulation. Simulated environments often lack the classic external disruptions and minor events that can overload and weaken the overall system. In addition, as mentioned above, situation awareness is uniquely developed through contact with actual environmental factors and practice with continuous situational assessment, which is critically important in managing issues during the course of an operation. Numerous studies have demonstrated fewer FDs, fewer communication issues, and improved decision-making among experienced surgeons and surgical teams [1, 5, 14, 16, 18–20]. Thus, a busier robotic surgery practice can improve situation awareness, reinforce team training, and decrease the cognitive workload on the team [3, 16, 20].

Lessons Learned/Personal Pearls

- The unique spatial configuration between the surgeon, patient, and console in robotic surgery places unique strains on the surgical team and situation awareness.
- Turnover time for cases involving robotic surgery may be longer and more variable than those that do not utilize this technology.
- Flow disruptions occur more often during robotic surgery, frequently caused by issues with coordination, communication, equipment, and training.
- Interventions to improve verbal and non-verbal communication, standardized training for the entire surgical team, workflow redeisgn, and experiential learning are crucial human factors tools to reduce errors and improve efficiency in robotic surgery.

References

1. Nyssen A-S, Blavier A. Verbal communication as a sign of adaptation in socio-technical systems: the case of robotic surgery. In: Proceedings of the 9th international conference on naturalistic decision making,, 2009, London, UK. Swindon: British Computer Society; 2009.
2. Zenati MA, Maron JK. Communication and teamwork failure as a barrier to robotic surgical safety. Paper presented at: 3rd joint workshop on new technologies for computer/robotic assisted surgery.
3. Randell R, Honey S, Alvarado N, et al. Embedding robotic surgery into routine practice and impacts on communication and decision making: a review of the experience of surgical teams. Cogn Tech Work. 2016;18:423–37.
4. Dulan G, Rege RV, Hogg DC, et al. Developing a comprehensive, proficiency-based training program for robotic surgery. Surgery. 2012;152(3):477–88.

5. Jain M, Fry BT, Hess LW, Anger JT, Gewertz BL, Catchpole K. Barriers to efficiency in robotic surgery: the resident effect. J Surg Res. 2016;205(2):296–304.
6. Brunckhorst O, Khan MS, Dasgupta P, Ahmed K. Effective non-technical skills are imperative to robot-assisted surgery. BJU Int. 2015;116(6):842–4.
7. Potretzke AM, Knight BA, Brockman JA, et al. The role of the assistant during robot-assisted partial nephrectomy: does experience matter? J Robot Surg. 2016;10(2):129–34.
8. Dexter F, Abouleish AE, Epstein RH, Whitten CW, Lubarsky DA. Use of operating room information system data to predict the impact of reducing turnover times on staffing costs. Anesth Analg. 2003;97(4):1119–26, table of contents.
9. Souders CP, Catchpole KR, Wood LN, et al. Reducing operating room turnover time for robotic surgery using a motor racing pit stop model. World J Surg. 2017;41(8):1943–9.
10. Friedman DM, Sokal SM, Chang Y, Berger DL. Increasing operating room efficiency through parallel processing. Ann Surg. 2006;243(1):10–4.
11. Rebuck DA, Zhao LC, Helfand BT, et al. Simple modifications in operating room processes to reduce the times and costs associated with robot-assisted laparoscopic radical prostatectomy. J Endourol. 2011;25(6):955–60.
12. Price M, Bates A, Clagett M. Improving efficiency and standardization in a robotics program: a quality improvement project. AORN J. 2018;108(6):652–60.
13. Cohen TN, Anger JT, Shamash K, et al. Discovering the barriers to efficient robotic operating room turnover time: perceptions vs. reality. J Robot Surg. 2020; https://doi.org/10.1007/s11701-020-01045-y.
14. Catchpole K, Perkins C, Bresee C, et al. Safety, efficiency and learning curves in robotic surgery: a human factors analysis. Surg Endosc. 2016;30(9):3749–61.
15. Catchpole KR, Hallett E, Curtis S, Mirchi T, Souders CP, Anger JT. Diagnosing barriers to safety and efficiency in robotic surgery. Ergonomics. 2018;61(1):26–39.
16. Allers JC, Hussein AA, Ahmad N, et al. Evaluation and impact of workflow interruptions during robot-assisted surgery. Urology. 2016;92:33–7.
17. Henaux PL, Michinov E, Rochat J, Hemon B, Jannin P, Riffaud L. Relationships between expertise, crew familiarity and surgical workflow disruptions: an observational study. World J Surg. 2019;43(2):431–8.
18. Tiferes J, Hussein AA, Bisantz A, et al. The loud surgeon behind the console: understanding team activities during robot-assisted surgery. J Surg Educ. 2016;73(3):504–12.
19. Ahmad N, Hussein AA, Cavuoto L, et al. Ambulatory movements, team dynamics and interactions during robot-assisted surgery. BJU Int. 2016;118(1):132–9.
20. Catchpole K, Bisantz A, Hallbeck MS, et al. Human factors in robotic assisted surgery: lessons from studies "in the wild". Appl Ergon. 2019;78:270–6.

Surgical Coaching 12

Jason C. Pradarelli, Caprice C. Greenberg, and Justin B. Dimick

What Is Surgical Coaching?

Surgical coaching is a meaningful strategy for surgeons' continuous professional development defined by a partnership between a surgeon and a coach. This partnership is not punitive but empowering for the surgeon who receives coaching—i.e., the "coachee." Surgical coaching focuses on individual performance improvement for surgeons at all talent and experience levels through structured, longitudinal, one-on-one reflections with a surgical coach.

Case Study

A highly funded endovascular surgeon, who was advancing to full professor, increasingly noted that her interactions with the operating room (OR) staff were contentious to the point of disrupting her operations. In her most recent case, a patient with a ruptured aortic aneurysm nearly died on the table because of an argument that transpired when the wrong stent grafts were opened on the back table. Given the complex, multidisciplinary nature of her cases, the surgeon requested that her Division Chief coach her by video recording her during an operation, reviewing the operative video with her, offering constructive feedback regarding her interactions with the OR team, and helping her set an action plan to improve those

J. C. Pradarelli (✉)
Department of Surgery, Brigham and Women's Hospital, Boston, MA, USA
e-mail: jpradarelli@partners.org

C. C. Greenberg
Department of Surgery, University of Wisconsin School of Medicine and Public Health, Madison, WI, USA

J. B. Dimick
Department of Surgery, Michigan Medicine, Ann Arbor, MI, USA

T. N. Cohen et al. (eds.), *Human Factors in Surgery*,
https://doi.org/10.1007/978-3-030-53127-0_12

relationships. By asking insightful questions, the Division Chief—i.e., her coach—helped the surgeon realize that her challenging interpersonal interactions were likely related to exhaustion from a high number of overnight calls, a consistently busy operative schedule, and several research commitments with ongoing clinical trials. Through guided self-reflection with her coach, she decided to scale back her call schedule and delegate certain research duties so that she could dedicate more attention to preparing the OR staff for her complex elective cases. The surgical coaching process helped her to improve her relationships with the OR staff as she was better able to plan and discuss cases with her team before stress arose during the operation itself.

Examples

To illustrate how surgical coaching facilitates surgical performance improvement, we expand on how practicing surgeons can engage with established surgical coaching programs. These examples demonstrate surgical coaching interactions using two different models for assessing a surgeon's performance: direct observation-based coaching and video-based coaching.

Direct Observation-Based Surgical Coaching

The Harvard Surgical Coaching for Operative Performance Enhancement (SCOPE) program is a surgical coaching program that utilizes direct observation as substrate for the coaching interactions. In SCOPE, practicing surgeons are paired with another surgeon at the same institution and assigned to either the "coach" or "coachee" role. Regardless of their role, all surgeons undergo a 3-hour coach training workshop to learn the core principles and practical skills of surgical coaching. These core principles—self-identified goals, collaborative analysis, constructive feedback, and action planning [1]—are grounded in the Wisconsin Surgical Coaching Framework (Fig. 12.1). The workshop leads surgeons through adopting the coaching mindset, applying coaching principles to a surgical context, and then practicing surgical coaching via video-based simulation (Fig. 12.2). The workshop and program are led by a multidisciplinary team of surgeons, a human factors organizational psychologist, and a professional coaching expert in the field of education.

In SCOPE, coach-coachee pairs follow a defined structure centered around an operation: preoperative goal-setting, intraoperative observation, and postoperative debriefing (Fig. 12.3). The coachee surgeon is expected to set their own goals related to topics that they want to learn, improve upon, or master. The coach is expected to facilitate the coachee's goal-setting by being an active listener, asking probing questions, and demonstrating empathy. For this example, let's suppose that the coachee's goal is to improve their communication and teamwork practices with the nursing and anesthesiology teams in the OR.

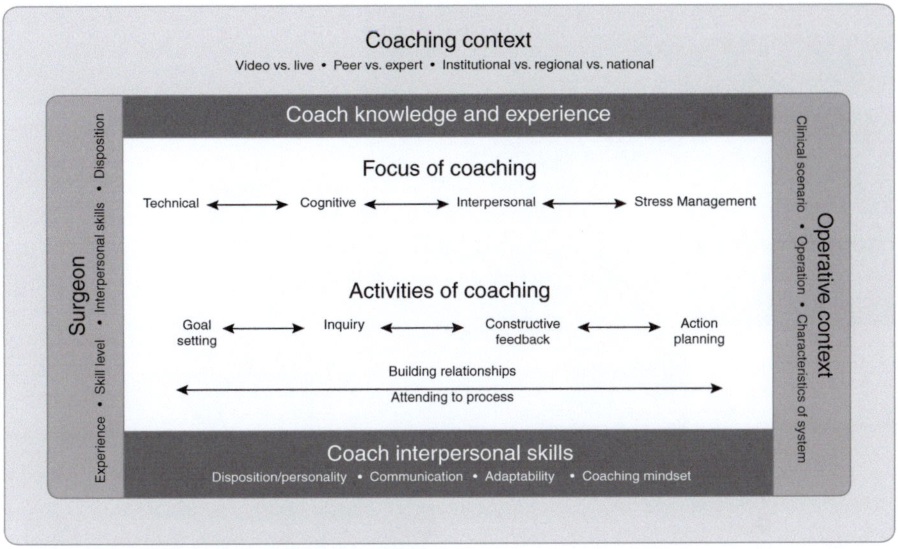

Fig. 12.1 Wisconsin Surgical Coaching Framework, 2016. (Source: Caprice Greenberg, MD, MPH)

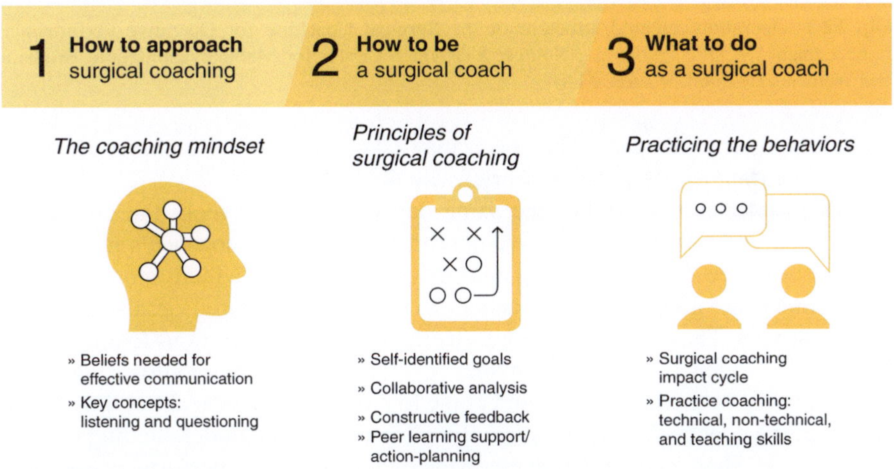
1 How to approach surgical coaching
2 How to be a surgical coach
3 What to do as a surgical coach
The coaching mindset
Principles of surgical coaching
Practicing the behaviors
» Beliefs needed for effective communication
» Key concepts: listening and questioning
» Self-identified goals
» Collaborative analysis
» Constructive feedback
» Peer learning support/ action-planning
» Surgical coaching impact cycle
» Practice coaching: technical, non-technical, and teaching skills

Fig. 12.2 Design of the introductory coaching workshop for the Surgical Coaching for Operative Performance Enhancement (SCOPE) program, 2018. (Source: Jason Pradarelli, MD, MS)

In the intraoperative phase of SCOPE, the coachee performs the operation as usual without the involvement of the coach. The coach observes but does not scrub into the case or intervene in any other way. They simply observe, focusing their observations primarily on the coachee's previously stated goals—in our example, on the coachee's communication behaviors and teamwork interactions with the

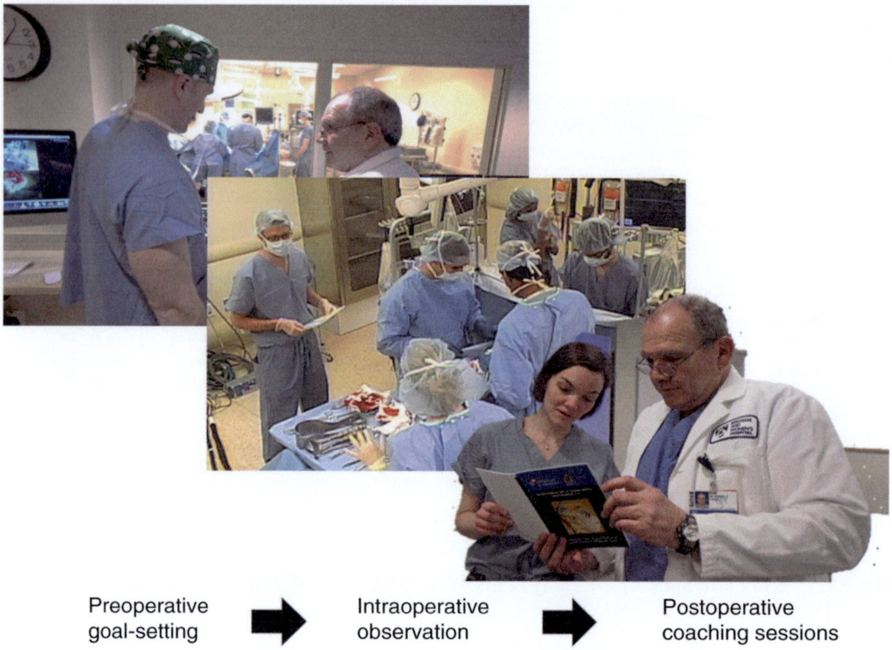

Fig. 12.3 Operation-centered structure of the Surgical Coaching for Operative Performance Enhancement (SCOPE) program. (Source: STRATUS Center for Medical Simulation, Brigham and Women's Hospital, Boston, MA)

multidisciplinary OR team. The coach may take notes on these observations for reference during a postoperative debrief with the coachee.

After the operation, either the same day or within a week, the coach and coachee sit down in a postoperative debrief to discuss the coachee's intraoperative performance. In this coaching interaction, the coach is a facilitator of discussion aimed at guiding the coachee toward reaching the goals they set preoperatively. The coach often begins using open-ended questions to understand the coachee's view of their performance. Collaborative analysis allows the coach to use inquiry to exchange ideas and come to a joint conclusion about the current reality of the coachee's performance. Based on this shared understanding of reality, the coach shares constructive feedback on the coachee's performance-related goals. For example, a coach might say, "I noticed that the anesthesiologist asked you a question about your progress in the case and you did not answer the question. It seems important to close the loop of communication with all team members so the patient can get the best care from the team. How did you view that interaction?" By delivering the feedback with a question, the coachee has an opportunity to reflect on the coach's observation and internalize the feedback. Finally, the coach guides the coachee to develop an action plan to continue pursuing the coachee's original goals or to develop new goals for improving their performance related to communication and teamwork in the OR. This cycle repeats itself longitudinally when the coach and coachee reassess interval progress and revisit the original goals at the next operation's preoperative goal-setting conversation.

Video-Based Surgical Coaching

Though based in the same coaching framework, the Wisconsin Surgical Coaching Program (WSCP) and the Michigan Bariatric Surgery Collaborative (MBSC) differ from the Harvard SCOPE program by utilizing a video-based coaching model. In WSCP and MBSC, coaching pairs are arranged within a statewide collaborative. Surgical coaches across the state also undergo a coach training workshop to learn foundational coaching principles. Surgeons are introduced to the performance domains of technical skills, cognitive non-technical skills, interpersonal non-technical skills, and stress management, although they can choose to focus their coaching discussions on any intraoperative performance topic. While the training is the same, the identification of coaches is different in Wisconsin and Michigan. In Wisconsin's initial program, coaches were identified by peer nomination based on both surgical skills and interpersonal characteristics known to enhance coach effectiveness. In contrast, the MBSC had ranked surgeons based on surgical skills ratings from peer review of intraoperative video; MBSC coaches were selected from among the surgeons with highest peer-rated surgical skills and best postoperative outcomes.

In a video-based coaching model, the basic structure still centers around an operation and follows the same coaching principles: goal-setting, collaborative analysis, feedback, and action planning in a longitudinal, iterative process. The key difference is that a video recording of the surgeon's operation is used to anchor the conversation (Fig. 12.4), rather than direct observation during a case. Surgeon participants record a video of any operation for which they want to receive coaching, and they have the option to send the video to their coach for review before meeting for a coaching session.

With the flexibility offered by video recording, coaches and coachees can schedule a coaching session at their convenience. The coaching session may be conducted locally at the coachee's institution, or at a neutral site such as a regional or national meeting. At existing society meetings, surgeons can block time with their coach, sparing the need to accommodate both surgeons' operating schedules during a regular work week. Although a "tele-coaching" model has yet to be tested, it may be possible to conduct a coaching session over the internet, utilizing screen-sharing technology so that both surgeons can view the operative video simultaneously from different locations. This question is actively under investigation. The coaching techniques used during the postoperative debrief in a video-based coaching model are the same techniques as described above for direct observation-based coaching.

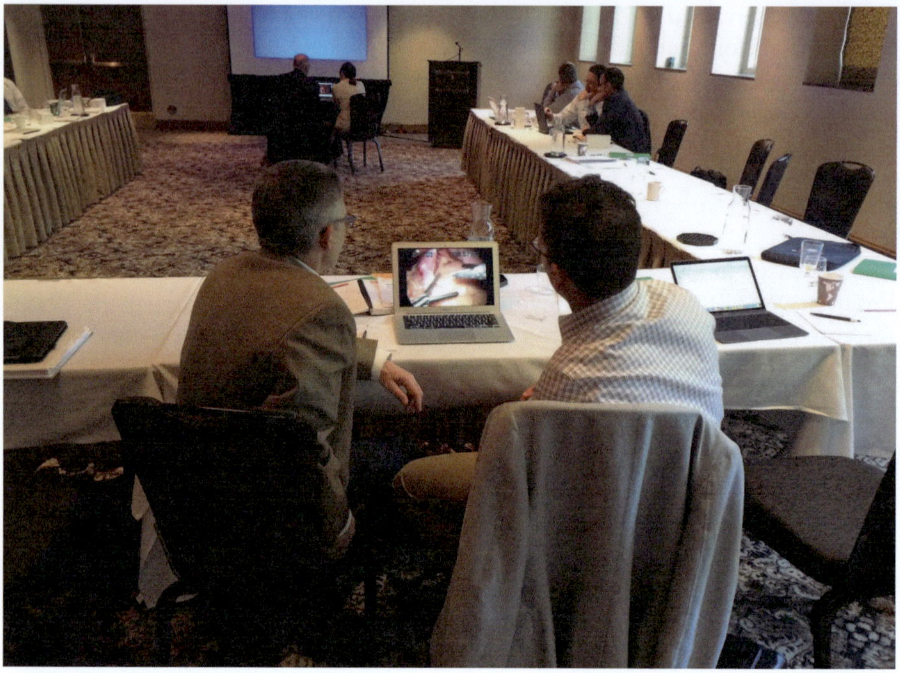

Fig. 12.4 Video-based peer surgical coaching in the Michigan Bariatric Surgery Collaborative (MBSC), 2016. (Source: Jason Pradarelli, MD, MS)

Surgical Coaching from a Human Factors Perspective

"Human factors" refers to the dynamic interaction between humans and the systems in which they function and interact. The human factors approach aims to optimize performance of individuals, teams, and systems. Surgeons and other individual healthcare providers can only perform their best when work activity is coupled with opportunities to analyze their own performance, receive and reflect on feedback about their performance, and adjust behaviors to improve their performance.

Although on initial glance, it may appear to be hyper-focused on the individual, surgical coaching aligns well with team-based and system-level interventions. The product of individualized coaching interactions between a surgeon and a coach has downstream effects on surgeons' teams and systems. As detailed in the earlier examples, surgical coaching provides a dedicated opportunity for surgeons to reflect on their clinical performance, acquire direct feedback, and receive assistance in planning for concrete behavior changes to improve the way they provide care to patients. This section will emphasize the range of patient care domains for which coaching can be incorporated to foster a culture of continuous performance improvement for individuals and their work environments.

Benefits of Surgical Coaching for Practicing Surgeons

Coaching can be used to guide individuals to improve any number of skills [2, 3]. Thus far, surgical coaching has primarily been applied in the context of clinical quality and patient safety. Existing evidence of coaching in surgery has focused on surgeons' technical and non-technical skills as intermediaries of quality and safety metrics. A commonly used assessment tool for technical skills is the Objective Structured Assessment of Technical Skills (OSATS), which measures operative skills like respect for tissue, time and motion, instrument handling, tissue exposure, and flow of the operation [1, 4, 5]. For non-technical skills, the Non-Technical Skills for Surgeons (NOTSS) system [6] offers a specific language to help surgeons improve their skill regarding the cognitive and social or interpersonal aspects of surgical performance [1, 5]. The cognitive skills in surgery refer to situation awareness and decision-making abilities in the OR; the social or interpersonal skills refer to a surgeon's leadership, communication, and teamwork abilities [6]. Better performance from surgeons on both technical skills [4] and non-technical skills [7] is associated with better patient outcomes, which is why surgical coaching programs focus on these domains of surgical performance.

In addition to practicing surgeons, video-based surgical coaching has also been studied among surgical trainees and medical students. Beyond technical skill improvements, a particularly interesting finding among surgical residents was improved insight into the assessment of their own performance after being coached [8]. While these findings have yet to be studied among practicing surgeons, they demonstrate valuable potential gains throughout the continuum of a surgeon's career.

Looking forward, coaching may realize additional important benefits for surgeons in other domains of their performance, including stress management, teaching skills, and operative efficiency, among others. Stress—and, in particular, management of a surgeon's stress—has been recognized as an important influence on both technical and non-technical skill performance. Multiple coaching sessions in the WSCP's first year dealt with recognition and mitigation of intraoperative stress for the participating surgeon [1]. Common sources of stress for surgeons include regular time pressures of the OR environment and the perception of poor assistance during a case. When teaching surgical trainees during an operation, surgeons may struggle with these key sources of stress; thus, coaching to improve specific teaching skills may coincide with improving stress management and prove to be beneficial to practicing surgeons.

By focusing on clinical skill improvements, such as decision-making and leadership of multidisciplinary teams, coaching could simultaneously enhance the efficiency of clinical operations. Direct observation and individualized feedback on a surgeon's operative flow may reduce OR resource utilization and costs. Similarly, coaching might help a surgeon identify opportunities to eliminate wasteful use of clinic resources as a sustainable way to enact cost savings.

One of the goals of surgical coaching is to empower practicing surgeons to take ownership of their own quality and performance improvement and to help make required continuing professional development more relevant to individual practice.

Importantly, surgical coaching also serves as a venue for relationship building among colleagues and encourages a collaborative learning approach. With burnout becoming a national priority for the surgeon workforce, surgical coaching also holds promise to address some of the underlying aspects of modern surgical practice that are associated with burnout.

Barriers to Implementing Surgical Coaching

Despite the myriad benefits to individual surgeons, logistical and cultural barriers present a challenge for widespread adoption of surgical coaching. Common sources of resistance for many professional development initiatives—limited time and financial constraints—also apply to surgical coaching. The Harvard SCOPE program exemplifies coaching that takes place within one's own institution, sparing the time and expense of traveling to conferences or to inconvenient off-site professional development events. Alternatively, the WSCP and MBSC programs offer examples for surgeons and surgical coaches who may participate in regional or national meetings, thus maximizing the value of these meetings. By adapting to surgeons' and coaches' preferences with on-site or off-site discussions, surgical coaching may create better value of professional development time for all parties involved.

The financial investment in surgical coaching can be mitigated by aligning interests with local organizations that could subsidize the costs of implementing a coaching program. For instance, when physicians continually work to improve their performance in a professionally satisfying environment, patient care and physician morale mutually benefit, reducing many risks that health insurers (e.g., Blue Cross Blue Shield of Michigan and the MBSC program) and malpractice insurers (e.g., CRICO and the Harvard SCOPE program) prefer to avoid. At individual institutions, funds invested in current continuing medical education activities of questionable value could be re-purposed for more meaningful opportunities such as surgical coaching. Leveraging creative partnerships with local funding sources can offset the costs of implementing coaching programs.

Finally, we must acknowledge surgical culture itself as an important—but not insurmountable—barrier to implementing surgical coaching. Early interviews with practicing surgeons about their perceptions and potential concerns about surgical coaching revealed three main cultural barriers: (i) perceived value of technical skill (assuming the coaching focused on technical skill improvements), (ii) concerns about image and authority, and (iii) loss of self-regulatory control [9]. In an invited commentary to this study, the authors emphasized that these three areas of concern align well with the basic principles of coaching, suggesting instead that coaching can actually support surgeons' professional priorities and that better education about the core principles of coaching is needed (Table 12.1) [10].

While recognizing that surgeons highly value competence and professional autonomy, these major areas of cultural concern can be addressed by clarifying the coaching model. (i) As described earlier, coaching may be applicable to all aspects of surgical performance, whether in the operating room or in a non-clinical context.

Table 12.1 Surgeon-identified barriers to surgical coaching and their counterarguments

Surgeons' concern	Description of surgeons' concern	Coaching principle/ Counterargument
Value of technical skill	Surgeons in academic practice feel that they have sufficient technical skill in their defined set of procedures and would rather concentrate on other areas of their career given limited time and energy for self-improvement.	1. Coaching may offer efficient approaches that can replace current ineffective approaches [8]. 2. Coaching may be applicable to all aspects of surgical performance (technical, non-technical) in the OR or any other clinical or academic setting [2].
Concerns about image and authority	The appearance of competence and expertise is critical given the responsibility and gravity associated with performing an operation.	1. Remove coaching from clinical setting as private, confidential interaction with a coach [8]. 2. Nonpunitive programs open to participants at all levels [1].
Loss of autonomy	Surgeons desire to maintain control over their learning agenda	1. Adherence to well-developed coaching principles of choice and voice, self-directed learning [3] 2. Develops capacity for self-assessment [8]

Adapted from Greenberg and Klingensmith [10]

Identifying performance goals that are meaningful to the individual surgeon is foundational to a coaching interaction, regardless if those goals are technical, non-technical, or even non-clinical. (ii) Surgical coaching is a nonpunitive form of professional development. Surgeons at all talent levels—including and especially high-performers—may benefit from coaching because the learning goals are tailored to the individual. Furthermore, the coaching interaction itself takes place outside of the OR in a private, confidential environment [10]. (iii) Coaching, by definition, empowers the individual surgeon to change behavior under their own will. Respecting a surgeon's autonomy and professional identify is an essential part of the coach training process. Thus, adhering to the core principles of coaching may enable surgeons to embrace surgical coaching as a powerful tool to improve performance while respecting their hard-earned professional identities.

Lessons Learned in Surgical Coaching

- From a human factors perspective, surgical coaching helps surgeons interact optimally with their teams in a complex, multidisciplinary patient care environment.
- The key behaviors of surgical coaching involve individualized goal-setting, collaborative analysis of the surgeon's performance with constructive feedback, and action planning to help the surgeon define concrete next steps to improve.
- Peer coaching requires that practicing surgeons put aside their typical hierarchical roles in educational activities to function as equal partners with other surgeons.

- Effective surgical coaches need to have a high level of emotional intelligence, excellent communication skills, and the respect of their peers.
- A coaching relationship involves listening and observing, asking insightful questions, inviting surgeons to reflect on their own behavior, and guiding surgeons to understand how to improve their own performance. Coaching is *not* directing, criticizing, pontificating, or giving in-the-moment advice to a surgeon.
- In contrast to group-oriented knowledge transmission with teaching and broad advice-giving with mentoring, coaching focuses on an individual's development of a specific skill, using self-reflection and exploratory techniques to motivate the surgeon to change behavior.
- Despite potential cultural concerns about surgeons' image, authority, and professional autonomy, surgical coaching done well may better align with surgeons' professional priorities than current approaches to continuing professional development and be a powerful tool to improve performance throughout a surgeon's career.

Disclosures
Dr. Pradarelli reports research grants from the Risk Management Foundation of the Harvard Medical Institutions, Inc., a part of Controlled Risk Insurance Company (CRICO), and from Johnson & Johnson Medical Devices and Diagnostics Global Services. Dr. Greenberg reports research grants from the National Institutes of Health (NIH), the Agency for Healthcare Research and Quality (AHRQ), and the Wisconsin Partnership Program. Dr. Greenberg is a consultant to Johnson & Johnson and is the co-founder and president of the Academy for Surgical Coaching. Dr. Dimick reports research grants from the NIH and AHRQ. Dr. Dimick is an equity owner of ArborMetrix.

References

1. Greenberg CC, Ghousseini HN, Pavuluri Quamme SR, Beasley HL, Frasier LL, Brys NA, Dombrowski JC, Wiegmann DA. A statewide surgical coaching program provides opportunity for continuous professional development. Ann Surg. 2018;267:868–73.
2. Greenberg CC, Ghousseini HN, Quamme SRP, Beasley HL, Wiegmann DA. Surgical coaching for individual performance improvement. Ann Surg. 2015;261:32–4.
3. Knight J. Better conversations: coaching ourselves and each other to be more credible, caring, and connected. Thousand Oaks: Corwin; 2016.
4. Birkmeyer JD, Finks JF, O'Reilly A, Oerline M, Carlin AM, Nunn AR, Dimick J, Banerjee M, Birkmeyer NJO. Surgical skill and complication rates after bariatric surgery. N Engl J Med. 2013;369:1434–42.
5. Pradarelli JC, Delisle M, Briggs A, Smink DS, Yule S. Identifying naturalistic coaching behavior among practicing surgeons in the operating room. Ann Surg. 2019; https://doi.org/10.1097/SLA.0000000000003368.

6. University of Aberdeen. The non-technical skills for surgeons (NOTSS) system handbook v1.2: structuring observation, rating and feedback of surgeons' behaviours in the operating theatre. Aberdeen: University of Aberdeen; 2006.
7. Cooper WO, Spain DA, Guillamondegui O, et al. Association of coworker reports about unprofessional behavior by surgeons with surgical complications in their patients. JAMA Surg. 2019;154(9):828–34.
8. Bonrath EM, Dedy NJ, Gordon LE, Grantcharov TP. Comprehensive surgical coaching enhances surgical skill in the operating room: a randomized controlled trial. Ann Surg. 2015;262:205–12.
9. Mutabdzic D, Mylopoulos M, Murnaghan ML, Patel P, Zilbert N, Seemann N, Regehr G, Moulton CA. Coaching surgeons: is culture limiting our ability to improve? Ann Surg. 2015;262:213–6.
10. Greenberg CC, Klingensmith ME. The continuum of coaching: opportunities for surgical improvement at all levels. Ann Surg. 2015;262:217–9.

Part IV

Specific Surgical Areas

Human Factors Considerations in Cardiac Surgery

13

Paul Frank, Michael Nurok, and Thor Sundt

What Is Cardiac Surgery?

Cardiac surgery requires multiple highly specialized teams of diverse backgrounds, education, and culture working in concert. Teamwork and communication are essential to achieving a successful outcome.

Case Scenario

A 73-year-old man presenting to the emergency department (ED) with severe chest and back pain at 2 am on a Sunday morning is found to have a type A aortic dissection. While waiting for the operating room (OR), he is started on a labetalol infusion through a peripheral IV. A transthoracic echo (TTE) shows an ejection fraction of 35% with severe aortic insufficiency and hypokinesis of the entire anterior wall. Given the emergency nature of the case, a cursory handoff between the ED and anesthesia teams was performed, confirming only the patient's name, age, and allergies.

The tired junior surgeon, who had just finished a heart transplant 2 hours earlier and is anxious about delaying the scheduled cases due to start in just a few hours, encourages the OR staff to prepare and drape the patient quickly. The scrub tech on call this evening usually assists ENT cases. The circulating nurse, who just started

P. Frank
Department of Anesthesiology, Cedars-Sinai Medical Center, Los Angeles, CA, USA

M. Nurok (✉)
Department of Surgery, Smidt Heart Institute, Cedars-Sinai Medical Center, Los Angeles, CA, USA
e-mail: michael.nurok@cshs.org

T. Sundt
Division of Cardiac Surgery, Corrigan Minehan Heart Center, Massachusetts General Hospital, Boston, MA, USA

T. N. Cohen et al. (eds.), *Human Factors in Surgery*,
https://doi.org/10.1007/978-3-030-53127-0_13

working at this institution 1 month ago, has never worked with this surgeon. The staff pulls instruments and sutures based on the only preference card they can find, which is for a different cardiac surgeon.

While the attending anesthesiologist is placing the transesophageal echo (TEE) probe, the patient's heart rate increases to 90 beats per minute. The resident starts a diltiazem drip through a newly placed central line, unaware that labetalol is running through a peripheral IV. Before the skin incision is made, the blood pressure drops to 44/27, and ST elevations are noted on rhythm strip. The surgeon cuts down on the femoral artery and vein. The anesthesiologist cannot visualize the venous guidewire in the inferior vena cava (IVC) on TEE. As she is communicating this to the surgeon, the surgeon's pager goes off—the intensive care unit (ICU) is calling about high chest tube output and new hypotension in the fresh heart transplant patient. After asking the ICU team to contact the on-call surgical resident, the surgeon advances the venous cannula over the guidewire without repositioning it. The cannula does not advance easily but is left in place as the patient's hypotension persists. Arterial cannulation is uneventful.

When the surgeon calls to initiate bypass, the perfusionist notices that an activated clotting time (ACT) sample has not been run. The anesthesiologist, who was discussing Saturday's football game with the circulating nurse, realizes she did not hear the surgeon ask for heparin administration. Heparin is administered and a norepinephrine drip initiated. Bypass is initiated after a satisfactory ACT is achieved but venous return is poor. The venous cannula must be removed and replaced, further delaying the repair.

Bypass time is prolonged, as the circulating nurse makes four separate trips to the core to obtain specific sutures and instruments requested by the surgeon. Upon returning from the core, the nurse trips on the bypass tubing and nearly falls into the sterile field. At 6 am, a new scrub tech and circulating nurse relieve their colleagues working the night shift. Unfortunately, the transition coincides with weaning and separation from bypass. The incoming team is unaware that this critical step is underway, and the surgeon delays weaning from bypass to orient them to the case.

The patient is weaned from bypass only after the second attempt and administration of high-dose infusions of epinephrine, dobutamine, and vasopressin. The anesthesiologist, exhausted after her third overnight case in the last 7 days, neglects to advise the ICU that the ventricular pacing cable has only been intermittently capturing, and that a skin lead is buried under a dressing. Thirty minutes after handoff to the ICU, the patient goes into a junctional rhythm with heart rate in the 20s. When the V lead fails to capture, new transcutaneous pacing pads are applied emergently, and transcutaneous pacing is initiated. Transvenous pacing is subsequently placed. The presence of a skin lead is not identified until the next morning.

Considerations in Cardiac Surgery

The complexity of cardiac surgical care has grown exponentially with the proliferation of life-sustaining interventions both in the operating room and ICU. These interventions are dynamic, complex, and critical to patient survival. The sheer amount of information and number of variables clinicians must manage and to which they must respond is staggering. For example, a patient in cardiogenic shock may have a temporary left and/or right ventricular assist device with specific flow and power settings, dependent on preload and sensitive to afterload. He or she may be on infusions of intravenous inotropes, vasopressors, or inhaled vasodilators, titrated to cardiac index and pulmonary arterial pressures measured off a pulmonary artery catheter. Echocardiogram may reveal clot in the ventricle or a malpositioned inflow cannula. All of these occur before the patient enters the OR.

Communication and Teamwork

More so than patients in any other surgical subspecialty, cardiac surgical patients are cared for by many teams. Referral pools for cardiac surgery include interventional and general cardiologists, pulmonologists, and thoracic and vascular surgeons, among others. Each will have different background and understanding of the elements critical to successful surgery, and accordingly, the necessary preoperative evaluation of patients and different recognition of "red flags." The surgical teams themselves are increasingly differentiated as development of techniques and technology accelerates, with "ventricular assist device/transplant" surgeons often distinct from "coronary revascularization" or "structural heart/valve" teams. Highly functional systems—particularly for complex problems—use a combined "Heart Team" approach where decisions about the best procedure(s) are made in an interdisciplinary setting.

In the operating room, the patient is cared for by the cardiac surgeon performing the operation, the cardiac anesthesiologist manages the patient's hemodynamics and guides the operation with TEE, the perfusionist manages the cardiopulmonary bypass circuit, and other devices like intra-aortic balloon pump, extracorporeal membrane oxygenation, and cell saver, and the nursing and surgical technologist staff ensure that all proper instrumentation and grafts are available. Information must be shared quickly and effectively among these teams.

After the operation, the patient will be taken to the ICU, where the critical care intensivists monitor the acute phase of the patient's recovery, often in collaboration with subspecialized cardiologists in mechanical circulatory support, transplantation, electrophysiology, or heart failure as well as consultants in nephrology, pulmonology, infectious diseases, or other fields. Not only must each team have a mastery of its own specialty, but it must also understand how their work fits into the larger puzzle that is the care of the critically ill patient. Information must be shared in an unambiguous manner with all appropriate individuals, and clear lines of decision making must be established. In the operating room and in the ICU, clear communication and teamwork are essential.

Given the complexity of the endeavor, it is not surprising that errors occur. Barach et al. observed 102 pediatric cardiac surgical procedures, monitoring for adverse events, which they classified as major or minor [1]. Major events were those that may have serious consequences, such as accidental extubation while placing the TEE probe, aortic laceration during sternotomy, and depletion of the portable oxygen cylinder during patient transport. Minor adverse events—those not expected to have serious consequences—included communication breakdown, delay in bed availability, and electrocautery not being plugged in. The number of major events per case increased with case complexity ($p = 0.013$) and duration ($p = 0.048$). Intriguingly, however, the number of minor events per case did not correlate with case complexity or duration. Rather, "[t]he large number of minor events seems to indicate an environment awash with distractions, interruptions, and miscommunications." Communication failures were the most common type of minor adverse event, accounting for 29% of all minor adverse events. These failures were most common during cardiopulmonary bypass and induction of anesthesia, two critical periods for patient safety.

Barach's finding that complex cardiac surgical procedures carry greater risk of major adverse events is intuitive and consistent with the concept of "normal accidents" in complex endeavors [2]. However, the finding of breakdown in communication regardless of the complexity and duration of the operation suggests rich opportunities for improvement in teamwork and communication. Additionally, the finding that lapses in these areas are common suggests the impact could be significant.

Similarly, Wiegmann et al. observed 31 cardiac surgical cases, recording and classifying disruptions in surgical flow [3]. A full 52% ($n = 178$) of disruptions arose from problems with teamwork and communication—issues such as premature administration of heparin, lack of administration of inotropes, and lack of familiarity with surgeon preferences by the perfusionist. Alarmingly, this study demonstrated a correlation between the frequency of teamwork and communication errors and the frequency of technical surgical errors ($p < 0.001$). The high frequency of lapses in communication observed in Wiegmann show that even routine communication intended to coordinate activities that occur with every cardiac surgical case can be fraught with errors.

OR personnel for a typical cardiac surgical case includes, at minimum, a surgeon and an assistant, scrub technician, anesthesiologist, perfusionist, and circulating nurse. The individuals filling each of these roles each have a different work schedule and demands on their time, and their assignments may change as emergencies or other urgent needs arise. Therefore, it is rare that a single OR team will work together exclusively or even primarily. It has been shown that the incidence of surgical flow disruptions and surgical errors was markedly higher in OR teams that did not work together regularly ($p < 0.001$) [4]. Teams that work together regularly are more familiar with one another. Over time, they develop an implicit understanding of individual roles within the larger team as well as a shared mental model of the task that allows them to anticipate each other's actions [5]. This familiarity and shared mental model improves coordination and efficiency, and it allows for improved problem-solving capability in dynamic situations. The fact that teams who work together more frequently perform better is intuitive. But ensuring that only familiar teams are assembled, especially in emergency circumstances, is impractical, and how to optimize scheduling and on-call demands to maintain consistent teams remains a challenge.

Information sharing is difficult enough when all members of the team are physically present in the same space, treating the same patient at the same time. The complexity of care of the cardiac surgical patient extends beyond the OR, however. The postoperative handoff entails a transfer of care between two groups of interdisciplinary teams. It requires multiple points of information sharing—anesthesiologist to intensivist, OR nurse to ICU nurse, and sometimes OR perfusionist to ICU perfusionist—each of which requires a succinct and effective summary of the patient's status and relevant medical history. Much has been written about handoffs and the need for complete and succinct information. The literature suggests that handoffs are often unstructured, fraught with omissions and competing tasks, missing key personnel, and prone to frequent interruption [5]. It should come as no surprise, then, that much information, including critical facts and tasks, are not transmitted during handoffs.

Given the importance of communication and teamwork and the inability to consistently schedule the same individuals to work together, it is critical to empower teams to organize and share information as efficiently as possible. Several modalities have been implemented to achieve this purpose. Preoperative briefings are structured but open-ended discussions involving all members of the operative team. These discussions usually occur before the patient enters the OR and allow teams to share information, ask questions, and share concerns [6]. For example, the perfusionist may ask the surgeon which cannulas will be needed for cardiopulmonary bypass, or the OR nurse may raise the concern that no blood products have been ordered. The shared discussion is most effective when every member of the team is empowered to share information and raise concerns.

After induction of anesthesia and draping of the patient, and just prior to incision, the preoperative time-out must occur. Unlike the preoperative briefing, this is a closed-ended checklist and is mandated by the Joint Commission. The time-out must confirm patient identity, procedure, laterality (if relevant), and patient allergies. Over time, other items have been added to the time-out, such as fire risk and instrument sterility. Each team within OR may also rely its own checklist in order to prevent overlooking critical items.

At the conclusion of the operation, a debriefing may take place. As with the preoperative briefing, the postoperative debriefing is an open-ended discussion among all team members, reviewing the case, what went well, and what did not. The intention is that teams will identify and focus on areas of improvement.

After leaving the OR, the patient is often taken to the ICU, where a handoff takes place. The potentially haphazard nature of this critical time for patient safety can be organized by implementation of structured communication. For example, the anesthesiologist signing out to the intensivist might always start the handoff with patient name, age, and procedure performed, followed by hemodynamic drips, device settings, blood products administered, and post-bypass TEE findings. The predictable and orderly nature of this type of structured communication will help prevent the provider of information—the anesthesiologist in this case—from neglecting important facts, while also helping the receiver of information—the intensivist in this case—know what information to expect and in what order.

Such highly structured information sharing and role assignment has already been successfully incorporated into other safety-critical industries such as Formula 1 racing and aviation. Catchpole et al. consulted with experts in Formula 1 racing and aviation to develop a new structured handoff from the OR to the ICU for congenital cardiac surgical patients. Highlights of the new paradigm include the following:

- The anesthesiologist is responsible for overall team coordination.
- There are three defined phases to the handoff (equipment handoff, information handoff, and discussion/plan).
- Only essential communication is allowed (first the anesthesiologist, then the surgeon).
- Checklists are used to prevent oversights.

In a prospective trial of the new paradigm comparing 23 usual handoffs and 27 handoffs guided by the new paradigm, there were reductions in technical errors (e.g., equipment not plugged in or key personnel absent), omissions of information (e.g., blood products, antibiotics), and duration of handoff [7].

Ineffective communication within and among teams unquestionably can harm patients. For information to be shared effectively, communication needs to be clear, open, organized, and succinct.

Physical Environment

As with any other specialized piece of equipment, the size and layout of the operating room should be designed as ergonomically as possible, with foremost consideration given to safe and successful completion of the task at hand. In many settings, the size and layout of operating rooms are not optimal for the task of cardiac surgery.

The complex and interdisciplinary nature of cardiac surgery necessitates the presence of more people and more equipment than in a non-cardiac operation. As a result, operating rooms can often become overcrowded and loud. The size of large equipment such as the TEE machine and the cardiopulmonary bypass machine, as well as bypass tubing and other cables snaking across the floor, can inhibit the safe and expeditious movement of personnel in the operating room. This poses a danger not only to staff, who may trip on tubing or hit their head on a low-hanging monitor, but also for the patient, for whom life-saving intervention may be delayed due to space constraints or providers unable to hear one another over background noise.

Palmer et al. observed 10 cardiac operations and documented disruptions to surgical flow. Over 10 cases, an astounding 1080 unique disruptions were recorded and organized into one of six categories [8]. The most common cause of flow disruption was the physical layout of the OR, accounting for 31% of disruptions. Issues with the physical layout of the OR include positioning of equipment (e.g., CPB machine), furniture (e.g., chairs), and permanent structures (e.g., doorways) that hinder the

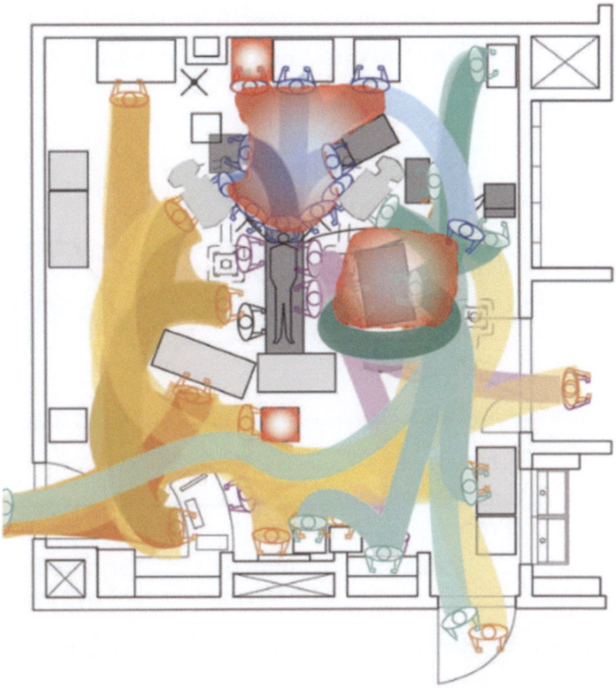

Fig. 13.1 Architectural flow diagram. Architectural plan indicating composite staff movement during the operative phase of observed procedures. The personnel are identified by a specific color (anesthesiologists are denoted in *blue*, surgeons in *purple*, nurses in *tan*, and perfusionists in *green*). Each representation of a person indicates locations they have traveled, not the total number of people involved in the surgery. The *density of the line color* indicates the magnitude of movement within the time period studied. *Red zones* indicate areas with a high density of flow disruptions. Used with permission. (Palmer et al. [8])

efficient movement of staff in and around the OR. Figure 13.1 shows the movement of OR personnel during the procedures observed in Palmer. Areas of high congestion are highlighted in red. The most congested areas in the OR are the head of the bed—the anesthesia workspace—and the perfusion area, where the CPB machine is located.

The second-most common cause of flow disruption encompassed the general milieu interruptions from common annoyances like phone calls, pagers, and shift changes [8]. When a phone rings or pager goes off, the circulating nurse or other OR staff usually stops their own work to answer it and relay information between the caller and recipient of the call, often the surgeon. Depending on the length and content of the call, there can be significant delay to the case as well as loss of the cognitive flow of the operation. The team may need to reacquaint itself in order to safely resume the procedure at hand.

A particularly tricky source of increased noise and distraction in the OR environment is that of side conversations and music. Some practitioners may find music helpful, and some find it distracting. Beyond that, there is the question of what kind of music and how loud it should be. Desires for music, or extraneous small talk, are sometimes context-dependent. Complicating matters is the fact that different team members have different cognitive workloads at different times during the operation. For example, during induction of anesthesia, the surgeon and perfusionist may feel free to discuss their vacation plans, while the anesthesiologist may desire quiet. Figure 13.2 shows a plot of cognitive workloads of various OR personnel throughout

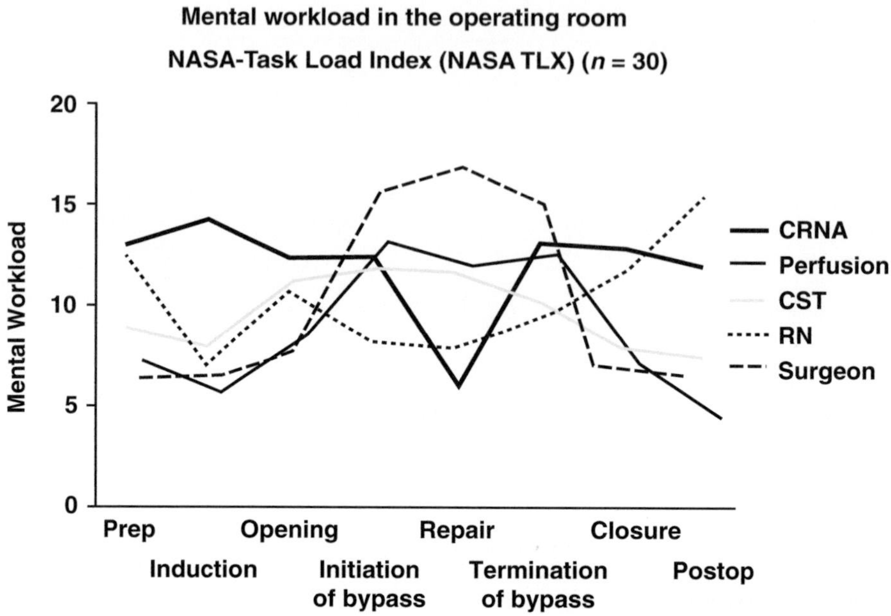

Fig. 13.2 Mental workload in the cardiac operating room. Mental workload in the cardiac surgery operating room varies across the cardiac surgery procedure for individual providers depending on task complexity and responsibilities. CRNA, certified registered nurse anesthetist; CST, certified surgical technologist; NASA, National Aeronautics and Space Administration; Postop, postoperative; Prep, surgical preparation; RN, registered nurse; TLX, Task Load Index. Used with permission. (Wahr et al. [5])

the phases of a cardiac operation [5]. Presumably, an individual with a low cognitive workload at a given time, such as the certified registered nurse anesthetist during bypass time, would be more amenable to music in the background or some small talk, whereas the surgeon would be less agreeable to background noise at that time.

Given the multitude of environmental challenges faced by large multidisciplinary cardiac surgical OR teams, many interventions have been suggested in order to eliminate the congested and boisterous nature of the OR. For example, staff changes for lunch breaks and changes of shift can be timed to occur during less critical parts of the operation, such as during skin closure instead of during initiation of bypass. Additionally, pagers and phones can be attended to by an appropriate individual who is not participating in the operation. These changes can be implemented relatively quickly and on a small scale, expanding over time as pilot programs prove successful. Other environmental factors, such as the size and configuration of the OR, as well as the size of some equipment, cannot be addressed in such an ad hoc fashion. Rather, these changes will come as departments and institutions make large capital investments in new facilities and equipment. It is important that stakeholders—namely the highly trained personnel who work in the ORs every day—have input into plans for new or renovated ORs.

A challenge for all team members is the proliferation of equipment and monitoring devices, which in isolation may serve beneficial purposes but in aggregate may add to cognitive workload and can serve as sources of distraction. For example, with the now routine use of TEE—especially prior to and at the time of separation from CPB—some programs have elected to distribute the cognitive workload and have a separate anesthesia team perform TEE while a primary team focuses on all other aspects of anesthetic management. Of course, some technology reduces cognitive workload, as has been the case with electronic record keeping and monitoring. In general, when technology is introduced into the OR, there should be consideration of and observation for unintended consequences. In addition, prior to introduction into the surgical environment, OR teams and hospital administrators should evaluate not only the purported salutatory effects of a piece of technology, but also the "overhead costs" of reduced physical space and increased cognitive workload that may accompany it.

Lessons Learned

- Cardiac surgery is a team endeavor. Successful outcomes require effective communication and coordination.
- Complete yet succinct handoffs between interdisciplinary teams are critical for patient safety.
- Each phase of a cardiac surgical procedure places differing sets of demands on different OR team members.
- Teams that work together frequently achieve better outcomes. Although this may be difficult to achieve, staff scheduling should be conducted with this in mind.
- The cardiac surgical OR is more crowded with personnel and equipment than a general OR. As such, the risk of excessive noise, traffic, and other sources of distraction is exacerbated.

References

1. Barach P, Johnson JK, Ahmad A, et al. A prospective observational study of human factors, adverse events, and patient outcomes in surgery for pediatric cardiac disease. J Thorac Cardiovasc Surg. 2008;136:1422–8.
2. Perrow C. Living with high-risk technologies. Princeton: Princeton University Press; 1999.
3. Wiegmann DA, ElBardissi AW, Dearani JA. Disruptions in surgical flow and their relationship to surgical errors: an exploratory investigation. Surgery. 2007;142:658–65.
4. ElBardissi AW, Wiegmann DA, Henrickson S. Identifying methods to improve heart surgery: an operative approach and strategy for implementation on an organizational level. Eur J Cardiothorac Surg. 2008;34:1027–33.
5. Wahr JA, Prager RJ, Abernathy JH, et al. Patient safety in the cardiac operating room: human factors and teamwork: a scientific statement from the American Heart Association. Circulation. 2013;128:1139–69.

6. Fann JI, Moffatt-Bruce SD, DiMaio JM, et al. Human factors and human nature in cardiothoracic surgery. Ann Thorac Surg. 2016;101:2059–66.
7. Catchpole K, De Leval M, McEwan A, et al. Patient handover from surgery to intensive care: using Formula 1 pit-stop and aviation models to improve patient safety and quality. Pediatr Anesth. 2007;17:470–8.
8. Palmer G, Abernathy JH, Swinton G. Realizing improved patient care through human-centered operating room design: a human factors methodology for observing flow disruptions in the cardiothoracic operating room. Anesthesiology. 2013;119:1066–77.

Applying a Human Factors Approach to Improve Patient Care in Colorectal Surgery

14

Karen N. Zaghiyan and Phillip R. Fleshner

What Is Colorectal Surgery?

Colorectal surgery involves abdominal and/or pelvic surgery involving the colon, rectum, or anus. Proctectomy involves removal of the rectum and is perhaps one of the most technically demanding operations within our subspecialty. When performed for rectal cancer, a total mesorectal excision (TME) is required to remove the lymph nodes en-block with the rectum. Total proctocolectomy with ileal pouch-anal anastomosis (IPAA) is the standard procedure for ulcerative colitis requiring surgery. These procedures, commonly performed through an open or laparoscopic approach, may be especially challenging in obese patients or males with a narrow pelvis. Transanal total mesorectal excision (TaTME) [1] and transanal ileal pouch-anal anastomosis (TaIPAA) [2] are innovative techniques whereby proctectomy is performed "bottom-up" through the anus. The advantage is that the transanal technique offers an in-line vantage point to the distal rectum—potentially improving surgical precision, oncologic outcomes, and functional outcomes while maintaining a minimally invasive approach. However, specialized training is required, and the learning curve is steep, with proficiency achieved at about 50 cases [3]. This procedure is frequently performed with two teams—one abdominal team and one tranasanal team—each with a unique attending surgeon, surgical assistant/resident, scrub technician, back table set up, and video tower. There are various unique risks to a transanal proctectomy including a higher risk of urethral injury and CO_2 air embolism [4]. The complexity of case set up and multiple steps and equipment also pose a greater opportunity for human error. As a result, there is a tremendous opportunity for human factors methods to improve patient outcomes.

K. N. Zaghiyan (✉) · P. R. Fleshner
Cedars-Sinai Medical Center, Los Angeles, CA, USA
e-mail: Karen.Zaghiyan@cshs.org

T. N. Cohen et al. (eds.), *Human Factors in Surgery*,
https://doi.org/10.1007/978-3-030-53127-0_14

Case Study

Two colorectal surgery cases involving TaTME or TaIPAA are presented to help understand how human factors can help achieve high quality care—one yielding poor outcomes and another where things go well.

When Things Can Go Wrong

A 52-year-old obese male with a T3N1 rectal cancer at 6 cm from the anal verge undergoes neoadjuvant chemoradiation and is referred for surgery. The patient seeks out a second-opinion surgical consultation 9 weeks post treatment. The case is presented at a multidisciplinary team conference; the patient is deemed an appropriate candidate for surgery and chooses to proceed with the second-opinion surgeon. The surgeon is trained and experienced in TaTME and recommends low anterior resection with coloanal anastomosis and diverting loop ileostomy using a two-team laparoscopic TaTME approach. In order to accommodate the patient within the standard 12-week post-radiation treatment window, the case is scheduled outside of the surgeon's block on a different operating floor. The assigned crew is unfamiliar with the operation or set up.

On the morning of surgery, the surgeon finds the scrub nurse scrambling to pull the requested instruments. The room is not ready. The regular 3D endoscope used for the transanal dissection is not available, so the surgeon agrees to use a different camera instead. The patient is finally brought to the operating theater after a 50-minute delay. The proctectomy, as anticipated, is challenging due to the low tumor and patient body habitus. The transanal surgeon encounters some bleeding during the anterior transanal dissection. The energy device, typically on standby in case of bleeding, is not in the room. There is only one scrub nurse assigned to the case and the circulating nurse has left the room to obtain a requested instrument. The anesthesiologist reports that he is unable to read an EKG rhythm. End-tidal carbon dioxide ($ETCO_2$) has suddenly decreased. He thinks the patient is in asystole. He calls a code-blue. The transanal surgeon releases insufflation in the rectum and asks the abdominal surgeon to do the same. He thinks this may be an air embolism. A bradycardic rhythm returns. The abdomen and pelvis are packed with gauze and the patient is transported to the intensive care unit.

Analysis: The complexity of TaTME requires not only surgical expertise but also a trained team including a circulator and scrub technician. The surgery also carries specific nuances such as the risk of air embolism that were not communicated by the surgeon to the team. In this case, the short post-radiation treatment window resulted in a hurried scheduling of the patient outside of the surgeon's block. The unfamiliarity of the staff with the case and setup yielded delays and surgeon frustration. Surgeon frustration potentially resulted in a lack of preoperative communication with the anesthesiologist. There were staffing shortages and lack of case preparation. The culmination of these factors resulted in a poor outcome for the patient.

When Things Go Well

A 26-year-old female with ulcerative colitis is scheduled for IPAA. A transanal approach is recommended for the proctectomy. The surgeon and assistant surgeon are trained in this technically challenging procedure. The nursing staff are familiar with the case, have all received specialized in-service training, and the case instruments are picked the night before. The anesthesiologist has previously worked with the surgeon and is aware of the case complexity and nuances. He is prepared and aware of the risk of air embolism. The surgeon checks in for the case early and communicates with the nursing and anesthesia staff to assure needed equipment and anticipated problems are addressed. He notifies the anesthesiologist of the plan for an intraoperative laparoscopic tranversus abdominis plane block and asks the anesthesiologist to watch for lidocaine toxicity during its administration. Two scrub technicians are assigned to the case: one for the transanal and one for the abdominal dissection. A two-team TaIPAA is performed. During the proctectomy phase of the operation, the abdominal and transanal dissections must connect to dismount the rectum. The two teams, each consisting of a surgeon, resident, and scrub technician, work simultaneously to dismount the rectum and deliver it transanally. The ileal pouch is created and passed down to the transanal surgeon. The scrub notices on the video monitor that the pouch appears twisted and points this out to the surgeons who immediately address the problem and reorient the pouch. The case completes without complication.

Analysis: In this case, not only were the surgeons trained and experienced in this challenging two-team TaIPAA but also the nursing staff were well trained and prepared. The case instruments were picked the evening prior to surgery and the operating theater was set up with the instruments and video towers placed according to the surgeon's specifications. The surgeon performed a preoperative briefing with both nursing and anesthesia staff to assure needed equipment and specific nuances regarding the case were addressed. The scrub felt comfortable with the interpersonal dynamics and voiced concern over the twisted pouch, which was immediately addressed by the operating teams. The smooth flow of surgery and case outcome were heavily influenced by the team dynamic, communication, and workflow.

How Can We Improve Complex Colorectal Surgery Using Human Factors Principles?

Colorectal surgery is a rapidly evolving field. Technological innovation has quickly transitioned the field from open surgery to one that has embraced a minimally invasive approach. With technological growth, the propulsion of technology into the operating theater has required surgeons and nursing staff to adapt and learn new techniques. The application of robotic technology in colorectal surgery is one example. While the application of robotic surgery has been thought of as generally safe and resulting in improved patient outcomes, various studies have identified workflow interruptions and communication errors during robotic surgery as factors influencing surgical delays and potentially adverse events [5, 6]. One study by Catchpole and colleagues [6] evaluated the rate of flow disruptions and operative duration in 89 robotic surgical cases across various surgical specialties such as Urology, Gynecology, and Cardiac Surgery. Factors influencing flow disruptions included various categories (Table 14.1). These disruptions may have been influenced by surgeon experience, surgical type, robot model, and patient characteristics. A mean of 9.62 flow disruptions per hour (95% CI 8.78–10.46) was predominantly caused by coordination, communication, equipment, and training problems. Operative duration and flow disruption rate varied with surgeon experience ($p = 0.039$ and $p < 0.001$, respectively), training cases ($p = 0.012$; $p = 0.007$), and surgical type (both $p < 0.001$). Flow disruption rates in the operative phase between patient arrival to the operating room and placement of ports were also sensitive to the robot model and patient age. This data suggests that complex robotic surgery increases the opportunity for technological failures and the need for communication among team members.

Table 14.1 Flow disruption definitions and examples

Categories	Definitions	Examples
Communication	Any miscommunication that impacts surgical progress	Surgeon on console unable to hear bedside assistant, who has to repeat communication
Coordination	Any lapse in teamwork to prepare for/conduct surgery that affects surgery flow	Surgeon always uses a specific piece of equipment, but staff fails to retrieve item prior to when it is needed during the surgery
External factors	Any interruption that is not relevant to the current case or surgery	Surgeon receives cell phone call or text message
Training	Any instruction by the attending surgeon to fellows, residents, or medical students	Surgeon instructing resident on where to place the ports
Equipment	Any equipment issue that affects the surgery progress	Robotic instrument expires and has to be changed during the case
Environmental	Any room condition that impacts the surgery progress	Music is too loud, making it difficult for staff to hear surgeon requests
Patient factors	Any patient characteristic that impedes efficient surgery progress	Obesity making port placement difficult
Surgeon decision making	Any surgeon pause to determine next surgical step	Surgeon states he/she wants to identify the ureter before moving forward
Instrument changes	Additional robotic surgery instrument changes	Surgeon changes the arms in which the grasper and bipolar are located and changes them back after testing the new arrangement

Adapted from Catchpole et al. [6]

Transanal total mesorectal excision is another form of surgical innovation in colorectal surgery. The procedure is technically challenging and carries a steep learning curve. From the surgical standpoint, creation of a proctectomy with bottom-up surgery introduces a new vantage point, but with opportunity for wrong plane dissection. Instruments are different than those used in standard laparoscopy (a transanal access platform and continuous insufflation management system are required and two video towers are required). Thus, this technique requires formal surgical training and carries a steep learning curve similar to robotic surgery. From a nursing standpoint, the operation carries multiple steps, increased number of instruments to supply the abdominal and tranasanal dissection, and two surgeons working simultaneously may require two scrub technicians. Nursing training and preparation is important. Furthermore, one of the unique nuances of TaTME is the risk of CO_2 air embolism. During TaTME, transanal high-pressure air insufflation can result in air embolism if venous bleeding is encountered during the anterolateral dissection of the rectum. Preoperative communication with anesthesia is necessary to alert and prepare for this risk.

In high-skill, complex operations such as in cardiac and transplant surgery, teams are created to help improve flow, communication, and outcomes. Within these teams, there is limited acceptance for team members to rotate in and out during an operation or to leave before the operation is complete. Teams also tend to be less hierarchical with more comfort and social equality among members. As a result, teams have better interpersonal communications and are able to learn the complex sequence of timed, coordinated procedures. The concept of a *team* is in contrast to a *crew*, which is composed of shift workers assembled on a rotating basis. A key aspect of a crew is the acceptance of new crewmembers who have limited experience as it is assumed that their limited procedure specific experience will have little negative impact on crew function. The downside, however, is that an exponential number of crew combinations are possible. This type of arrangement may be acceptable in common, low-risk operations, but not in tense situations or technically demanding operations [6]. In a study evaluating this concept, surgical procedures were assigned a novel team familiarity score (FS), defined as the sum of the number of times that each possible pair of the team had worked together during the previous 6 months divided by the number of possible combinations of pairs in the team [7]. FS was significantly associated with type and urgency of the procedure with the least familiar teams involved in emergency aortic procedures. FS was strongly associated with length of procedure but not length of stay or complication rates. A systematic review of minimally invasive surgery cases evaluating the role of non-technical skills noted that fixed teams improved teamwork and patient safety across studies, while deficient planning and poor teamwork were found to obstruct workflow and increase errors [8]. TaTME is a technically demanding operation high in technology and requires such fixed teams to operate well.

Unfortunately, in the first case presented, the patient was added onto the surgical schedule separate from the surgeon's typical operating block. As a result, an untrained crew was assigned to the case rather than the trained team that the surgeon was familiar with. In addition, the surgeon expected the surgical setup and flow to run as if his typical team was working alongside him. It is understandable that at times, the team may be dismantled. In these cases, the surgeon can step up and take the initiative to train the available staff about the surgical nuances of a case. The surgeon coming in earlier than planned or connecting with the operating staff on the day prior to surgery to alert them about the technical nuances may have helped ease the unfamiliarity of the case, improve team communication, reduce team hierarchy, and allows a more collaborative approach to improve the outcome of the case. Better communication prior to the day of surgery may have also helped assure appropriate staffing.

The concept of a human factors approach may be novel in surgery but is standard in the aviation industry [9]. This culture change in aviation occurred in the 1970s when several tragic accidents resulted in the realization that the technical skills of piloting an aircraft were insufficient to ensure safety; accidents were occurring for reasons beyond the pilot's skillset. Crew Resource Management (CRM) was developed in aviation to address non-technical skills. Adoption of a less hierarchical framework in the operating room, adoption of a blame-free culture of error management, use of crewmember debriefings and checklists, and crew performance measurements are some examples of CRM that can be applied to the operating theater. The World Health Organization surgical safety checklist was created with CRM principles in mind and has been shown to significantly reduce surgical morbidity and mortality. While the utility of a surgical time-out has become universally accepted, adoption of briefing and debriefing has lagged behind in surgical culture. In order for appropriate briefings to occur, the surgeon, anesthesiologist, circulator, and scrub should meet in the operating room before the patient is brought in. Each member discusses points that are important to them. For example, the surgeon mentions whether the procedure is standard or if there are any special needs, the circulator would identify any medication on the back table, the scrub would assure that needed equipment are on the field or in the room, and the anesthesiologist would ask if there are any specific problems or concerns to be aware of. This type of briefing has been adopted in the Kaiser Permanente healthcare system [10]. A debriefing would then occur at the end of the case, whereby blood loss, complications, wound class, and factors that went right and wrong are discussed (Table 14.2).

In the second case, the team was trained and familiar with the operation, and the anesthesiologist had also previously worked with the surgeon. The group met before surgery to discuss specifics and case nuances. The scrub felt comfortable communicating concern over the twisted pouch as there was little hierarchical structure. These factors all contributed to the superior outcome in this case.

Table 14.2 Example of a surgical briefing for transanal total mesorectal excision

Surgeon	Circulator	Scrub	Anesthesia
ID patient Realistic time estimate Desired position Expected blood loss Special equipment (e.g., flexible sigmoidoscopy) Special needs (matching of transanal and abdominal insufflation pressures) Anticipated problems (risk of air embolism) Any special intraoperative risks (e.g., bleeding—have vessel sealer available) Special medications on the field (indocyanine green for fluorescence angiography; local anesthetic for TAP block)	ID patient Allergies Verify dose of local anesthetic for block Verify that preoperative multimodal analgesia medications have been administered Verify preoperative subcutaneous heparin administered Verify blood available if needed	Verify all instruments opened or available Any instrument missing Any special instrument you may need	Type of anesthesia being used (plan to use rapid sequence in a patient with bowel obstruction) Ask if any problem should be anticipated Any special medication for pain control Confirm if surgeon doing TAP block or anesthesia Discuss plan to hold lidocaine drip used in the multimodal analgesia protocol due to patient history of cardiac arrhythmia

TAP transversus abdominis plane block

Lessons Learned/Personal Pearls

- Novel colorectal procedures like transanal total mesorectal excision may require complex operative setup and pose unique coordination and communication challenges.
- Less hierarchical teams that work together frequently during complex cases are preferable to crews who are composed of rotating shift members.
- When untrained crew members cannot be avoided, surgeons can take an active role in training and communicating with staff prior to an operation to ensure safety and efficiency.
- In addition to a surgical time-out, adoption of briefing and debriefing time with the surgeon, anesthesiologist, circulating nurse, and scrub technician before and after the case will facilitate discussion on expected blood loss, complications, or other potential challenges.

References

1. Atallah S, Albert M, Monsor JR. Critical concepts and important anatomic landmarks encountered during transanal total mesorectal excision (taTME): toward the mastery of a new operation for rectal cancer surgery. Tech Coloproctol. 2016;20:483–94.
2. Zaghiyan K, Warusavitarne J, Spinelli A, Chandrasinghe P, Di Candido F, Fleshner P. Technical variations and feasibility of transanal ileal-pouch anal anastomosis for ulcerative colitis and inflammatory bowel disease unclassified across continents. Tech Coloproctol. 2018;22:867–73.

3. Lee L, Kelly J, Nassif GJ, deBeche-Adams TC, Albert MR, Monson JRT. Defining the learning curve for transanal total mesorectal excision for rectal adenocarcinoma. Surg Endosc. 2020;34(4):1534–42. https://doi.org/10.1007/s00464-018-6360-4.
4. Dickson EA, et al. Carbon dioxide embolism associated with transanal total mesorectal excision surgery: a report from the international registries. Dis Colon Rectum. 2019;62:794–801.
5. Allers JC, et al. Evaluation and impact of workflow interruptions during robotic-assisted surgery. Urology. 2016;92:33–7.
6. Catchpole K, et al. Safety, efficiency and learning curves in robotic surgery: a human factors analysis. Surg Endosc. 2016;30:3749–61.
7. Powezka K, Normahani P, Standfield NJ, Jaffer U. A novel team Familiarity Score for operating teams is a predictor of length of a procedure – a retrospective Bayesian analysis. J Vas Surg. 2020;71(3):959–66. https://doi.org/10.1016/j.jvs.2019.03.085.
8. Gjeraa K, Spanager L, Konge L, Petersen RH, Ostergaard D. Non-technical skills in minimally invasive surgery teams: a systematic review. Surg Endosc. 2016;30:5185–99.
9. Wakeman D, Langham MR Jr. Creating a safer operating room: groups, team dynamics and crew resource management principles. Semin Pediatr Surg. 2018;27:107–13.
10. Leonard M, Graham S, Bonacum D. The human factor: the critical importance of effective teamwork and communication in providing safe care. Qual Saf Health Care. 2004;13(Suppl 1):i85–90.

Identifying Opportunities to Improve Processes in Emergency General Surgery

15

Mehreen Kisat and Ali Salim

Overview of Emergency General Surgery

The American Association for the Surgery of Trauma and the American College of Surgeons Committee on Trauma defined emergency general surgery (EGS) as a field in 2003. In the United States, EGS constitutes 7% of all hospital admissions and 850,000 EGS operations are performed every year [1, 2]. A recent study from the National Inpatient Sample defined seven emergency general surgery procedures, which account for 80% of the operative EGS burden [3]. These seven procedures include partial colectomy, small bowel resection, cholecystectomy, peptic ulcer disease, lysis of adhesions, appendectomy, and laparotomy. EGS patients are a unique subset of patients with higher rates of postoperative complications, mortality, readmissions, and care discontinuity (Fig. 15.1) [4].

Case Study

Case #1

A 70-year-old male presented to the emergency department (ED) with complaints of abdominal pain for 48 hours. A CT scan was obtained in the ED, which showed free air and fluid likely due to a small bowel perforation. The emergency general surgery (EGS) team was consulted. Upon evaluation, the patient was in septic shock with peritonitis on physical exam. The patient was taken to the operating room (OR) urgently for an exploratory laparotomy. A safety pause that included all of the team

M. Kisat
Brigham and Women's Hospital, Boston, MA, USA

A. Salim (✉)
Harvard Medical School, Brigham and Woman's Hospital, Boston, MA, USA
e-mail: asalim1@bwh.harvard.edu

T. N. Cohen et al. (eds.), *Human Factors in Surgery*,
https://doi.org/10.1007/978-3-030-53127-0_15

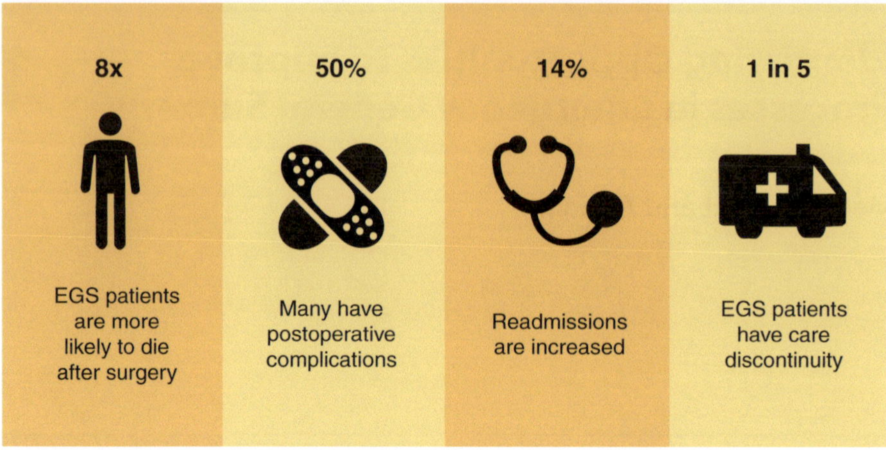

Fig. 15.1 Summary of emergency general surgery outcomes. (Reference: PMID: 29657721)

members in the operating room (surgery, anesthesia, scrub, circulator) was conducted before the surgical incision. The team was unable to tell whether the patient had received pre-operative antibiotics in the ED or not. A decision was therefore made to administer antibiotics. A laparotomy was performed and there was significant contamination of the abdomen due to a small bowel perforation. The patient continued to be hemodynamically unstable with escalating vasopressor requirements. This was not communicated clearly between the surgery and the anesthesia team. A bowel resection and anastomosis was performed. The patient received 4 units of packed red blood cells and 2 units of Fresh Frozen Plasma (FFP), even though blood loss was noted to be minimal by the surgery team. At the end of the surgery, the patient had improved clinically from a hemodynamic standpoint, but still had metabolic acidosis and a base deficit. It was determined that the patient needed to go to the intensive care unit (ICU) postoperatively. However, the circulating nurse did not anticipate this and had requested a floor bed instead of an ICU bed. The team waited in the OR for the next 60 minutes while an ICU bed was arranged, and the patient was then transferred to the ICU.

Analysis: There was a lack of communication between the ED team and OR team regarding pre-operative antibiotics. Then the patient's hemodynamic instability was attributed to blood loss and the surgery and anesthesia teams did not discuss the need for blood transfusions. The surgery team did not communicate the patient's postoperative disposition to the circulating nurse causing a delay in transfer to the ICU.

Case #2

The EGS service was consulted on a patient with choledocholithiasis for cholecystectomy during hospital admission. The patient had already undergone an endoscopic retrograde cholangiopancreatography by the gastroenterology team, which revealed multiple stones in the common bile duct. The patient was evaluated and the surgery team recommended a cholecystectomy. An appropriate sign out was performed between the medicine and surgery team before proceeding to the operating room. This included discussion of the need for any additional work-up for pre-op risk stratification, timing of surgery to determine NPO status, and if and when prophylactic anticoagulation should be held. In the operating room, during the safety pause, the possibility of conversion to an open surgery was discussed as the patient had a history of a previous hysterectomy and right colectomy. The surgery team discussed the necessary surgical instruments and retractors that would be needed in the event of an open operation. The circulating nurse made arrangements for the open cholecystectomy tray to be in the operating room. The team also discussed that the patient will be transferring to the surgery service postoperatively and a bed request for a bed on the surgery floor was established. Intraoperatively, there were significant adhesions and the critical view of safety for laparoscopic cholecystectomy could not be obtained and the decision to convert to an open operation was made. The surgery team communicated this with the anesthesia team. All the necessary equipment for an open cholecystectomy was in the room. After the conclusion of the operation, the patient was extubated and transferred to the recovery area. The patient went to the surgical floor postoperatively.

Analysis: Inpatient consultations require coordination and communication between the primary service and the EGS team for pre-op risk stratification, NPO status, and prophylactic anticoagulation. The surgery team discussed the plan for conversion to an open operation early and all the necessary equipment was present in the room. The disposition of the patient postoperatively was clarified and necessary arrangements were made.

Discussion of the Topic Including Human Factors

Institutional cultural norms and infrequent communication between the team members in the operating room can compromise a patient's safety in the operating room [5]. Implementation of the World Health Organization Surgical Safety Checklist (WHO SSC) has improved multidisciplinary communication practices and reduced morbidity and mortality in surgical settings [6–8]. This concept is borrowed from principles studied in the airline industry. The role of the checklist is to improve the completion of critical tasks, which have the potential of increasing risk or be life threatening if missed, at points where the detection of missed task is still possible [8]. The WHO Surgical Safety Checklist has three components to it. The first part occurs before the induction of anesthesia and is initiated by the anesthesia team and includes confirmation of the patient's identity, procedure, and consent and site marking. The second part occurs before skin incision and is initiated by the surgery team. It focuses on introduction of all team members by name and role, patient's identity, procedure and site of incision, and prophylactic antibiotics. The surgery, anesthesia, and nursing teams voice any anticipated critical events at this stage. The third part occurs before the patient leaves the operating room and is initiated by the nursing team and includes confirmation of the name of the procedure, completion of count, and specimen labeling [9]. The WHO SCC should be implemented 100% of the time in the operating room.

In addition to the checklist tools, team huddle strategies in which everyone on the team pauses and focuses their attention on a common task has been shown to improve communication between the different team members [10]. None of these tools had previously been examined or tailored to the need of EGS.

Approximately 3 million patients are admitted to US hospitals each year for EGS diagnoses [2, 11]. EGS patients are a unique surgical population who are at higher risk of morbidity and mortality. Patients who undergo an EGS operation are more likely to die compared to patients who have the same operation on an elective basis [12–14]. Approximately 50% of the patients undergoing emergency general surgery develop a postoperative complication [15]. Additionally, 15% of the patients are readmitted to the hospital within 30 days of their index operation [16]. Identification of the seven procedures, which account for 80% of procedures, deaths, complications, and costs has been vital in establishing EGS benchmarks [3]. This work has enabled us to understand the factors causing high morbidity and mortality in EGS patients and develop interventions to improve them. We conducted a retrospective cohort study of all adult patients who underwent EGS at two tertiary academic hospitals using the American College of Surgeons-National Surgical Quality Improvement Project database. We demonstrated that emergency general surgery is independently associated with high rates of intraoperative blood product transfusion. EGS patients were twice as likely to receive high-intraoperative pRBC use and three times more likely to receive high-intraoperative FFP use [12]. This work enabled us to identify modifiable factors contributing to the excess morbidity in EGS patients.

Based on this work, our division developed an evidence-based surgical safety tool aimed at encouraging the use of huddle strategies focused on modifiable factors unique to the EGS surgical subspecialty. The EGS communication tool works as an adjunct to the WHO SCC. Our communication tool was created through three phases: (1) identification of modifiable huddle points, (2) pilot testing, and (3) implementation of the tool in the OR. After demonstrating the feasibility of the EGS communication tool, we implemented it into all the operating rooms at our institution, and it is physically posted on the OR wall next to the WHO SCC in each OR [17] (Fig. 15.2).

In our practice, just before the surgical incision, in addition to the use of the standard WHO SCC, the EGS team acknowledges if the case is classified as an EGS procedure and verbalizes the anticipated postoperative disposition of the patient. Additionally, all the team members are encouraged to call a team huddle to discuss any concerns at any time. Use of the EGS communication tool in case #1 could have potentially prevented unnecessary blood transfusion in the patient by prompting the surgery and anesthesia team to have a conversation regarding the need for blood

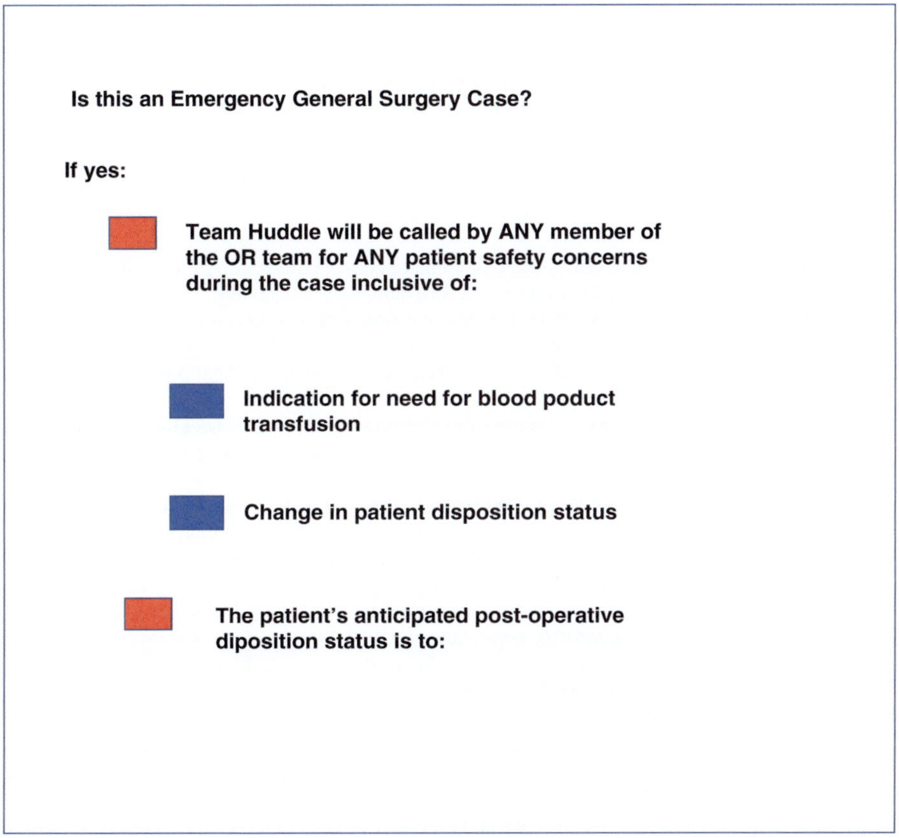

Fig. 15.2 The EGS communication tool (Reference: PMID 29907223)

transfusion. Additionally, even though the postoperative disposition might have been obvious to the surgery team, this was not translated to the OR circulating nurse. Discussing the potential postoperative disposition of the patient at the beginning of the case would have prevented the delay in transfer to the ICU. Future work will identify the long-term effects of this tool implementation on EGS patient morbidity and mortality.

Lessons Learned

- EGS patients are a vulnerable patient population. It is important to recognize that EGS patients are at increased risk of morbidity and mortality compared to patients undergoing the same operation on an elective basis.
- An EGS communication tool can potentially improve intraoperative communication and patient safety in this population.

References

1. Becher RD, Davis KA, Rotondo MF, Coimbra R. Ongoing evolution of emergency general surgery as a surgical subspecialty. J Am Coll Surg. 2018;226:194–200. https://doi.org/10.1016/j.jamcollsurg.2017.10.014.
2. Gale SC, Shafi S, Dombrovskiy VY, Arumugam D, Crystal JS. The public health burden of emergency general surgery in the United States: a 10-year analysis of the Nationwide Inpatient Sample—2001 to 2010. J Trauma Acute Care Surg. 2014;77:202–8. https://doi.org/10.1097/TA.0000000000000362.
3. Scott JW, et al. Use of National Burden to define operative emergency general surgery. JAMA Surg. 2016;151:e160480. https://doi.org/10.1001/jamasurg.2016.0480.
4. Lyu HG, Najjar P, Havens JM. Past, present, and future of emergency general surgery in the USA. Acute Med Surg. 2018;5:119–22. https://doi.org/10.1002/ams2.327.
5. Kim FJ, et al. Current issues in patient safety in surgery: a review. Patient Saf Surg. 2015;9:26. https://doi.org/10.1186/s13037-015-0067-4.
6. Russ S, et al. Measuring variation in use of the WHO surgical safety checklist in the operating room: a multicenter prospective cross-sectional study. J Am Coll Surg. 2015;220:1–11.e14. https://doi.org/10.1016/j.jamcollsurg.2014.09.021.
7. Treadwell JR, Lucas S, Tsou AY. Surgical checklists: a systematic review of impacts and implementation. BMJ Qual Saf. 2014;23:299–318. https://doi.org/10.1136/bmjqs-2012-001797.
8. Haynes AB, et al. A surgical safety checklist to reduce morbidity and mortality in a global population. N Engl J Med. 2009;360:491–9. https://doi.org/10.1056/NEJMsa0810119.
9. Weiser TG, et al. Perspectives in quality: designing the WHO Surgical Safety Checklist. Int J Qual Health Care. 2010;22:365–70. https://doi.org/10.1093/intqhc/mzq039.
10. Glymph DC, et al. Healthcare utilizing deliberate discussion linking events (HUDDLE): a systematic review. AANA J. 2015;83:183–8.
11. Havens JM, et al. Explaining the excess morbidity of emergency general surgery: packed red blood cell and fresh frozen plasma transfusion practices are associated with major complications in nonmassively transfused patients. Am J Surg. 2016;211:656–663 e654. https://doi.org/10.1016/j.amjsurg.2015.11.031.
12. Havens JM, et al. The excess morbidity and mortality of emergency general surgery. J Trauma Acute Care Surg. 2015;78:306–11. https://doi.org/10.1097/TA.0000000000000517.
13. Ingraham AM, et al. Comparison of hospital performance in nonemergency versus emergency colorectal operations at 142 hospitals. J Am Coll Surg. 2010;210:155–65. https://doi.org/10.1016/j.jamcollsurg.2009.10.016.
14. Ingraham AM, Cohen ME, Raval MV, Ko CY, Nathens AB. Comparison of hospital performance in emergency versus elective general surgery operations at 198 hospitals. J Am Coll Surg. 2011;212:20–28.e21. https://doi.org/10.1016/j.jamcollsurg.2010.09.026.
15. Patel SS, et al. Elective versus emergency surgery for ulcerative colitis: a National Surgical Quality Improvement Program analysis. Am J Surg. 2013;205:333–7, discussion 337–338. https://doi.org/10.1016/j.amjsurg.2012.10.014.
16. Havens JM, et al. Defining rates and risk factors for readmissions following emergency general surgery. JAMA Surg. 2016;151:330–6. https://doi.org/10.1001/jamasurg.2015.4056.
17. Columbus AB, et al. An evidence-based intraoperative communication tool for emergency general surgery: a pilot study. J Surg Res. 2018;228:281–9. https://doi.org/10.1016/j.jss.2018.03.007.

Human Factors in Surgical Oncology

16

Jessica S. Crystal and Alexandra Gangi

What Is Surgical Oncology?

Surgical oncology is the area of surgery that focuses on the management of patients with cancer. The effective practice of this complex specialty goes beyond the confines of the operating room (OR) and involves a multidisciplinary approach to the prevention, diagnosis, treatment, and long-term follow-up of these patients. The effective implementation of these practices requires a multidisciplinary team composed of surgical oncologists, medical oncologists, radiation oncologists, pathologists, radiologists, anesthesiologists, nurses, dieticians, physical therapists, technicians, pharmacists, palliative care physicians, among many other members of the medical community (Fig. 16.1). The goal of care is to prolong survival and alleviate suffering, while limiting the morbidity of administered treatments.

Case Study

Case 1 A 45-year-old female was found to have abnormal calcifications in the left breast. Diagnostic mammogram and ultrasound confirmed this finding. The lesion was stereotactically biopsied and a clip was placed at the biopsy site. Pathologic evaluation showed a triple-negative (estrogen receptor [ER], progesterone receptor (PR), human epidermal growth factor receptor 2 [Her2/neu] negative), infiltrating ductal carcinoma. The patient had no clinical evidence of axillary nodal disease, and given her diagnosis, she was then taken for a segmental mastectomy with sentinel lymph node biopsy. The localized area was resected, and the margins were incorrectly labeled prior to going for pathologic assessment. The final pathology showed residual tumor in the segment labeled "lateral margin," but this was actually the

J. S. Crystal (✉) · A. Gangi
Surgical Oncology, Cedars-Sinai Medical Center, Los Angeles, CA, USA

T. N. Cohen et al. (eds.), *Human Factors in Surgery*,
https://doi.org/10.1007/978-3-030-53127-0_16

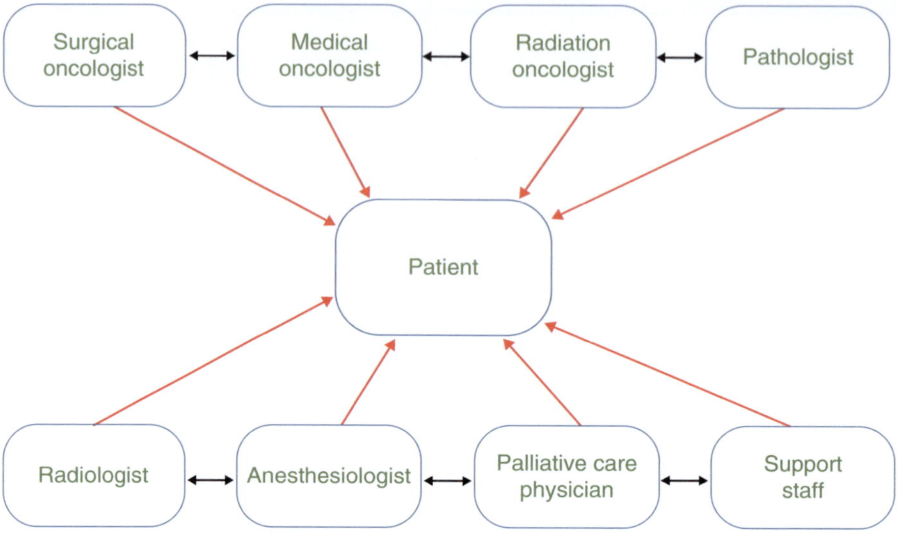

Fig. 16.1 Flowchart of multidisciplinary team

medial margin. The patient was small breasted and the need for re-excision resulted in a large defect that was aesthetically unpleasing. The final pathology showed a triple-negative breast cancer measuring 1.3 cm in size with no evidence of nodal disease. The additional surgery delayed the start of adjuvant chemotherapy and radiation treatment. The patient developed a local recurrence 2 years later and required a completion mastectomy and additional systemic therapy.

Analysis: Excellent communication is imperative to management of cancer. When the pathologists reviewed the specimen, the segmental mastectomy looked similar on all sides and was not clearly labeled. Clear labeling and communication between the surgeon, nursing staff, technologists, and pathologists to appropriately analyze the specimen are necessary. Unfortunately, this error had far-reaching adverse effects, including the need for additional surgery, poor cosmetic outcomes that were potentially avoidable, delay of adjuvant therapy, and potentially a local recurrence because the appropriate margin was not excised. In turn, this small problem can unfortunately play a large role in the outcomes of these patients.

Case 2 A 52-year-old male was found to have a low rectal mass on colonoscopy. Diagnostic workup showed what appeared to be a T3N0 rectal cancer. The patient's case was discussed at the institution's multidisciplinary tumor board conference, and it was decided that the best course of action would be to proceed with neoadjuvant chemotherapy and radiation prior to surgical resection. The patient received three cycles of folinic acid, fluorouracil, and oxaliplatin (FOLFOX), which was stopped early due to grade 3 toxicities, including sensory neuropathy and neutropenia. The patient also completed radiation therapy. Repeat imaging showed partial response of the tumor to neoadjuvant therapy. The patient's case was again discussed at the multidisciplinary tumor board and the decision was made to proceed with surgery. The patient was taken to the operating room for a robotic assisted low anterior resection. As is standard in many cases, a surgical stapler was used to perform the resection and anastomosis. However, the stapler used in this particular case had expired and misfired. The anastomosis "donuts" were not intact, and there was a positive leak test. The anastomosis was oversewn and a diverting ileostomy was created. Despite oversewing of the anastomosis and diversion, the patient's postoperative course was complicated by an anastomotic leak, requiring a return to the OR with resection of the anastomosis and placement of drains. The patient subsequently had a complicated hospital course and developed an abscess and required prolonged antibiotics. Additionally, he had persistently high output from the ileostomy, resulting in dehydration and electrolyte abnormalities. Unfortunately, the final pathology came back showing evidence of lymph node invasion (4/18) and residual disease in the rectum, but radial, proximal, and distal margins were negative. Due to the complicated postoperative course, adjuvant chemotherapy was delayed. On imaging 1 year postoperatively, the patient was found to have metastatic liver lesions. Despite trials of chemotherapy, the patient succumbed to the disease the following year.

Analysis: Management of patients with cancer is complex and requires a multidisciplinary team approach to provide excellent goal-directed and evidence-based care. The operative complexity for many cancer cases is quite high and often requires high levels of intraoperative judgment, especially in the setting of a stapler misfire. Therefore, these cases should be performed by individuals with specialized training to perform these procedures safely and to the standards set out by the oncologic community.

Applying Human Factors Concepts to Improve Surgical Oncology

When looking at the field of surgical oncology, it is quite similar to other fields of surgery; however, the pace at which treatments change in the field of oncology is much more rapid, and the complex treatment paradigms often require many different modalities provided by physicians of different specialties. This includes a combination of treatments, including surgery, systemic therapy (chemotherapy, targeted therapy, immunotherapy), and/or radiation therapy. The decision of whether or not to perform an operation or treat with any other modalities, or the timing of treatment, should not be taken lightly, as many of these therapies unfortunately have their own morbidities. Furthermore, management of cancer patients is a long-term process. Many therapies are given over months to years, and only provide full impact when treatment is given in its entirety and on a timely basis. Following completion of treatment, surveillance is required to watch for local, regional, and distant recurrence, and this process requires longer-term follow-up when compared to follow-up in some other surgical sub-specialties. Given that the estimated number of new cancer cases diagnosed in 2019 is approximately 1.7 million and the fact that cancer is the second most common cause of death in the US, exceeded only by heart disease, evaluating human factors to improve outcomes in these patients is essential [1].

Communication

Due to the complexity associated with surgical oncology, it is not surprising that communication issues represent one of the more common challenges experienced by team members. In a 2003 study, researchers evaluated and improved communication effectiveness during patient care rounds in a surgical oncology intensive care unit (ICU) [2]. In this study, researchers developed a survey to evaluate how well team members (residents and nurses) understood the goals of therapy. During the pre-intervention period, less than 10% of the team members understood the daily goals of therapy and the daily tasks to be completed. In an effort to improve understanding, the authors developed a daily goals form designed to facilitate communication by requiring the care team to communicate and define the goals for the day. The daily goals form was completed during rounds on each patient, was signed by either the fellow or attending physician, and subsequently passed on to the nurse. After implementation of the goals form, over 95% of the team members reported understanding the daily goals. Moreover, after the intervention was implemented, ICU length of stay decreased significantly from an average of 2.2 days to 1.1 days [2].

Training and Skill Development

The complexity of oncology surgery has been recognized in the scientific community and should be performed by those with the appropriate expertise and specialized training. Evidence for this includes a systematic review performed by Bilimoria et al., which showed that in 25 out of 27 studies reviewed, specialized surgeons had better outcomes for cancer surgery than nonspecialized surgeons. This included improved mortality, long-term survival, and lower recurrence, in 6 out of 10, 20 out of 27, and 6 out of 7 studies, respectively [3]. This was also shown by the study by Skinner et al., in which patients operated on by surgical oncologists had improved 5-year survival of 86% compared to 79% for patients treated by nonspecialized surgeons, even after controlling for both hospital and surgeon volume, as well as hospital, age, stage, and race [4]. These outcomes are likely a result of the treating physicians having been trained to routinely perform risk benefit analysis for particular cancer types and having a familiarity with navigating multimodality treatment plans and new paradigm shifts in care, which often include advanced techniques or new therapies. Of the many technologic advances adopted are the application of minimally invasive techniques, including laparoscopic and robotic surgeries, to oncologic operations. These techniques add another layer of complexity to the case, as advanced training is needed for both the surgeon and the rest of the operating room staff to operate and maintain these devices. The benefit of these minimally invasive techniques for management of some cancers has been shown in some studies to be related to the use of these advanced technologies; however, these findings are not consistent in all studies. In Markar and Lagergren's review of surgical and surgeon-related factors in managing esophageal cancer, they noted that the long-term survival benefits are actually more reflective of the surgeon's skill-related factors than the different surgical approach to the case [5].

Training and skill development can be challenging for surgical oncology trainees. Notably, Lewis and colleagues maintain that there has been a decline in the training opportunities available for cancer surgery, primarily due to the limit on trainee work hours, developments in nonsurgical treatments for cancer, and innovations in surgical technology [6]. The authors argue that because of these limitations, surgical oncologists must augment their training with nontraditional methods. One unique approach has involved the application of virtual reality (VR) simulation, namely in laparoscopic surgical training. VR simulation allows trainees to practice realistic procedures in a simulated and controlled environment. Moreover, previous research has demonstrated that VR simulation can significantly improve skills acquisition for surgical trainees [6].

Coordination of Care and Multidisciplinary Teamwork

Another component of the highly specialized center is its coordination of care, partly as a result of regularly scheduled multidisciplinary meetings. In fact, these conferences are a requirement for the National Cancer Institute Comprehensive Cancer Center designation and the Commission on Cancer designation [7]. This is a result of research showing that these conferences positively impact the quality of care, as was shown in a systematic review of 27 articles, which found that patients who were discussed at these meetings were more likely to be accurately and completely staged preoperatively and have received neoadjuvant and adjuvant treatment. Despite these benefits, the study unfortunately did not actually show any improvement in survival [8]. While less specialized and low-volume centers may have these meetings, their physicians are less likely to attend them [9].

Efficiency

Crucial to the management of patients with cancer is the timing of diagnosis and treatment. When systemic issues result in a delay in diagnosis or treatment, as occurred in the aforementioned examples, there can be a profound impact on the patient. For instance, looking at the diagnostic side, the timing of delivery of a specimen from the operating room to the pathologist can be critical to assessing the molecular data of the specimen. The "cold ischemia time" from when the specimen is removed from the patient to when it is fixed in pathology is associated with systems factors, including communication from the physician to the OR staff about what the specimen is, the transport time between the OR and the pathology suite, and appropriate handoff and transmission of that information to the pathologist analyzing the specimen. The importance of this handoff has been recognized in breast cancer regarding HER2/neu by the American Society of Clinical Oncology/College of American Pathologists (ASCO-CAP), who have strongly recommended fixation of tissue within 1 hour [10].

Unfortunately, delays in care and timing of surgery result in adverse outcomes, as shown by Mateo et al. in the National Cancer Database (NCDB) retrospective review of patients with noninflammatory, invasive breast cancer who had a decrease in survival after delay in surgical treatment [11]. Delays in chemotherapy are similarly as troublesome, as shown in a meta-analysis of over 15,000 patients in 10 studies, in which every 4-week delay in adjuvant chemotherapy after surgery resulted in a 14% decrease in overall survival [12]. Given that the current treatment for most malignancies involves multiple modalities, having repeat delays in care may be compounded and have a significant impact on the outcomes of these patients.

Case Volume

Another factor associated with improved outcomes in cancer patients is the surgical case volume of the hospital at which the patient is treated. This is particularly the case when dealing with complex surgeries like a pancreaticoduodenectomy, as shown in the national cohort study by Birkmeyer et al. In this study, Medicare patients who were cared for at centers with operative volume ranging from very low (<1/y) to high (5+/y) volumes were evaluated. Higher mortality rates were found to be significantly associated with very-low- and low-volume hospital centers compared to high-volume hospitals (12% and 16%, respectively, vs. 4%, $p < 0.001$) [13]. Other examples of the association of hospital volume to outcomes are shown in Table 16.1. It is likely that these outcomes result from multiple factors, including, but not limited to, better multidisciplinary care and pre- and postoperative supports.

The improved outcomes in high-volume centers extend to other treatment modalities as well, including the administration of single- and multi-agent chemotherapy and radiation. David et al. showed improved median overall survival in patients receiving multi-agent chemotherapy and radiotherapy for pancreatic cancer at high-volume compared to low-volume centers (14.3 months versus 11.2 months, respectively [$P < 0.001$]) and academic versus nonacademic centers (12.1 months versus 10.8 months, respectively [$P < .001$]) [24].

Patient Factors and Communication

In discussing these scenarios, it is important to acknowledge that the factors impacting surgical oncology do not just relate to the physicians' role in care but may also have to do with patient issues. For instance, delay in initiation of chemotherapy in patients has been found to occur more commonly in patients with comorbidities or

Table 16.1. Table of hospital volume studies

Study	Year	Volume Categories	LVH (# cases)	HVH (# cases)	Study period	# of patients	Data source	Surgery type	Results
Sosa et al. [14]	1998	Tertiles	4	20	1990–1995	1,236	Maryland Health Services Cost Review Commission Database	Pancreas resection (no specification)	The relative risk (RR) of in-hospital death after pancreatic resection was 19.3 and 8 at the LVH and MVH, respectively, versus the HVH, (95% confidence interval [CI] 5.5–68.1).
Simunovic et al. [15]	1999	Tertiles	22	42	1988–1995	842	Canadian Institute for Health Information	Pancreas resection (no specification)	Likelihood of postoperative death was higher in LVH and MVH centers than in HVH centers (odds ratio (OR) 5.1 and 4.5, respectively; ($p < 0.01$ for both).
Birkmeyer et al. [16]	2002	Quintiles	1	17	1994–1999	10,530	National Medicare claims database and the Nationwide Inpatient Sample	Pancreas resection (no specification)	Absolute differences in adjusted mortality rates between VLVH and VHVH ranged from over 12% for pancreatic resection, (16.3% vs. 3.8%).
Ho and Heslin [17]	2003	Quartile	1	10	1988–1998	6,652	California and Florida discharge database	PD	Patients undergoing PD in HVH (4–9/year) had a significantly lower mortality rate than in LVH (1 /year) (OR = 0.70, $P = .01$), and even lower in VHVH performing 10+ procedures per year (OR = 0.34, $p < 0.001$).
Urbach et al. [18]	2003	Quartile	3	25	1994–1999	686	Canadian Institute for Health Information	PD	If the 75% of patients treated at the LVHs had instead been treated at the HVHs, the annual number of lives potentially saved would have been 6(95% CI, 1–11) for PD.

(continued)

Table 16.1. (continued)

Study	Year	Volume Categories	LVH (# cases)	HVH (# cases)	Study period	# of patients	Data source	Surgery type	Results
Birkmeyer et al. [19]	2007	Tertiles	2	8	1992–2002	855	SEER–Medicare	Pancreas resection (no specification)	Absolute differences in 5-year survival probability rates between LVHs and HVHs for pancreas resection was 5% (10.8% vs. 15.9%)
Balzano et al. [20]	2008	Quartiles	5	89	2003	1,576	Bureau of Statistics, Italian Ministry of Health	PD	Increasing hospital volume was associated with a significantly reduced mortality rate: 12.4% (adjusted OR 1.000) for LVH, 7.8% (OR 0.611) for MVH, 5.9% (OR 0.466) for HVH and 2.6% (OR 0.208) for VHVH.
Bilimoria et al. [21]	2008	Tertiles	1	10	1994–1999	13,107	National Cancer Database	PD, DP, TP	The adjusted perioperative mortality at the LVH versus HVH was 2.26 versus a long-term hazard ratio of 1.13.
Gasper et al. [22]	2009	sextile	5	50	2000–2004	3,010	California discharge database	Pancreas resection (no specification)	The risk-adjusted mortality rate at the HVH was lowest compared to the LVH centers at 1.5% versus 5.6%, respectively.
Teh et al. [23]	2009	sextile	2	36	1988–2003	103,222	Nationwide Inpatient Sample	PD, DP, TP	After adjusting for other confounders, the odds of in-hospital mortality for PD, DP, and TP in those 65 years or older were lower by 4.78-, 3.84-, and 2.60-fold, respectively, when comparing the HVH with LVH.

PD pancreaticoduodenectomy, *DP* distal pancreatectomy, *TP* total pancreatectomy, *VLVH* very-low-volume hospital, L*VH* low-volume hospital, *MVH* medium-volume hospital, *HVH* High-volume hospital, *VHVH* very-high-volume hospital with poor access to care [25]. This is further emphasized by Shapiro et al.'s retrospective study of early-stage, resectable pancreatic adenocarcinoma in the Surveillance, Epidemiology, and End Results (SEER) database [26]. In the study, the gold standard of care for patients with this stage of cancer was resection, and the resection rate varied depending on sociodemographic characteristics (race, ethnicity, marital status, geographic location, and insurance status). This study also showed that cancer-specific survival differed by geographic location, even after adjusting for other relevant malignancy-related factors, with patients in the Pacific West (Hazard Ratio (HR) for death = 0.706; 95% confidence interval (CI), 0.628–0.793), Northeast (HR for death = 0.766; 95% CI, 0.667–0.879), and Midwest (HR for death = 0.765; 95% CI, 0.640–0.913) having improved survival compared to those in the Southeast (all $p < 0.001$) [26]. Other disparities affecting outcomes in cancer patients are associated with race, as shown in the analysis of the SEER database by Shah et al., in which there were fewer surgeries offered and performed in African Americans compared with Caucasians (adjusted odds ratio (aOR) 0.88, 95% CI 0.82–0.95; aOR 0.83, 95% CI 0.76–0.91, respectively). Even when surgery was recommended, African Americans were less likely to actually undergo surgery for their cancer (aOR 0.73, 95% CI 0.64–0.85) [27]. Additionally, in another study using the Netherlands Cancer Registry, patients were more likely to start their therapy later if they were older than 65 years of age, had emergency resection, and/or had a prolonged postoperative admission [28].

As previously mentioned, the surgical oncologist participates in the care of the patient beyond the operating room. This involves participation in the prevention/detection of the disease and the subsequent surveillance of the patient for development of local and distant recurrences as early as possible so they have potential to still be controlled. An important component of surveillance is compliance with the diagnostic measures to detect disease. As shown in Standeven et al.'s retrospective study of stage II/III colorectal cancer patients who completed cancer treatment, compliance is imperfect, and only 49% of the patients complied with all of the diagnostic tools. This is despite the fact that majority of the recurrences (88.4%) were being detected using these tests [29]. The imperfect compliance is a result of factors on multiple levels. This includes policy-level barriers like not having an organized screening program or testing procedure. Provider-level barriers are a result of inadequate counselling by providers, long wait times for tests and patient visits, inadequate screening of risk factors, and poor communication. Patient factors include level of education, literacy, income, perception, and cultural values, among other factors [30].

Levinson and colleagues discussed effective ways to develop physician communication skills for patient-centered care [31]. Patient-centered communication has been found to improve clinical outcomes in cancer management by having a positive impact on many of the factors described earlier, such as adherence to recommended treatment and self-management of chronic disease [32]. In an effort to improve communication, Nestel and colleagues developed an advanced surgical oncology communication program [33]. The program involves focusing on patient-centered communication and interprofessional communication. Patient-centered communication training involves a review of patient assessment skills like technical elements of communication and structural approaches to interactions. Trainees would learn how to collect biomedical and psychosocial information, explore patient feelings and expectations, acknowledge the patient/family's context, and develop a shared management plan. Additionally, they would learn how to address barriers to patient-centered communication, practice information-giving skills (e.g., explaining risks, describing treatments, and delivering bad news). Interprofessional communication training involves reviewing strategies for conducting effective handoffs, patient assessments, and patient care planning. Trainees would also learn how to run team meetings, review human factors, perform individual and team appraisals, and deal with team conflict.

Overall, bringing attention to human factors issues associated with surgical oncology is important in improving the outcomes of patients. Providers and patients need to continue to learn from their experiences to optimize their future.

Lessons Learned

- Management of cancer patients requires the interaction and collaboration of multiple medical professionals.
- Effective care is achieved at highly specialized, high-volume centers, who are skilled at managing these complex patients.
- Human factors issues associated with timing of diagnosis and treatment and compliance to screening and surveillance contribute to patient outcomes.
- Surgeons specializing in surgical oncology have expertise in providing multimodality treatment plans and adapting to new paradigm shifts in care, including advanced techniques or new therapies.
- Trainees may be able to improve their patient-centered communication and interprofessional communication via educational programs.

References

1. Siegel RL, Miller KD, Jemal DVM. A. Cancer statistics, 2019. CA Cancer J Clin. 2019;69:7.
2. Pronovost P, Berenholtz S, Dorman T, Lipsett PA, Simmonds T, Haraden C. Improving communication in the ICU using daily goals. J Crit Care. 2003;18(2):71–5.
3. Bilimoria KY, Phillips JD, Rock CE, et al. Effect of surgeon training, specialization, and experience on outcomes for cancer surgery: a systematic review of the literature. Ann Surg Oncol. 2009;16:1799–808.
4. Skinner KA, Helsper JT, Deapen D, Ye W, Sposto R. Breast cancer: do specialists make a difference? Ann Surg Oncol. 2003;10(6):606–15.
5. Markar SR, Lagergren J. Surgical and surgeon-related factors related to long-term survival in esophageal cancer: a review. Ann Surg Oncol. 2020;27(3):718–23.
6. Lewis TM, Aggarwal R, Rajaretnam N, Grantcharov TP, Darzi A. Training in surgical oncology–the role of VR simulation. Surg Oncol. 2011;20(3):134–9.

7. Cancer Program Standards. Ensuring patient-centered care. Chicago: American College of Surgeons; 2015.
8. Pillay B, Wootten AC, Crowe H, Corcoran N, Tran B, Bowden P, Crowe J, Costello AJ. The impact of multidisciplinary team meetings on patient assessment, management and outcomes in oncology settings: a systematic review of the literature. Cancer Treat Rev. 2016;42:56–72.
9. Scher KS, Tisnado DM, Rose DE, Adams JL, Ko CY, Malin JL, Ganz PA, Kahn KL. Physician and practice characteristics influencing tumor board attendance: results from the provider survey of the Los Angeles Women's Health Study. J Oncol Pract. 2011;7(2):103–10.
10. Compton CC, Averbook BJ. Precision surgical oncology? The treasure is in the tissue. Bull Am Coll Surg. 2018;103:30.
11. Mateo AM, Mazor AM, Obeid E, Daly JM, Sigurdson ER, Handorf EA, DeMora L, Aggon AA, Bleicher RJ. Time to surgery and the impact of delay in the non-neoadjuvant setting on triple-negative breast cancers and other phenotypes. Ann Surg Oncol. 2019;27:1679.
12. Biagi JJ, Raphael MJ, Mackillop WJ, Kong W, King WD, Booth CM. Association between time to initiation of adjuvant chemotherapy and survival in colorectal cancer: a systematic review and meta-analysis. JAMA. 2011;305(22):2335–42.
13. Birkmeyer JD, Finlayson SR, Tosteson AN, Sharp SM, Warshaw AL, Fisher ES. Effect of hospital volume on in-hospital mortality with pancreaticoduodenectomy. Surgery. 1999;125(3):250 6.
14. Sosa JA, Bowman HM, Gordon TA, Bass EB, Yeo CJ, Lillemoe KD, et al. Importance of hospital volume in the overall management of pancreatic cancer. Ann Surg. 1998;228:429–38.
15. Simunovic M, To T, Theriault M, Langer B. Relation between hospital surgical volume and outcome for pancreatic resection for neoplasm in a publicly funded health care system. CMAJ. 1999;160:643–8.
16. Birkmeyer JD, Siewers AE, Finlayson EV, Stukel TA, Lucas FL, Batista I, Welch HG, Wennberg DE. Hospital volume and surgical mortality in the United States. N Engl J Med. 2002;346(15):1128–37.
17. Ho V, Heslin MJ. Effect of hospital volume and experience on in-hospital mortality for pancreaticoduodenectomy. Ann Surg. 2003;237:509–14.
18. Urbach DR, Bell CM, Austin PC. Differences in operative mortality between high- and low-volume hospitals in Ontario for 5 major surgical procedures: estimating the number of lives potentially saved through regionalization. CMAJ. 2003;168:1409–14.
19. Birkmeyer JD, Sun Y, Wong SL, Stukel TA. Hospital volume and late survival after cancer surgery. Ann Surg. 2007;245(5):777–83.
20. Balzano G, Zerbi A, Capretti G, Rocchetti S, Capitanio V, Di Carlo V. Effect of hospital volume on outcome of pancreaticoduodenectomy in Italy. Br J Surg. 2008;95(3):357–62.
21. Bilimoria KY, Bentrem DJ, Feinglass JM, Stewart AK, Winchester DP, Talamonti MS, Ko CY. Directing surgical quality improvement initiatives: comparison of perioperative mortality and long-term survival for cancer surgery. J Clin Oncol. 2008;26(28):4626–33.
22. Gasper WJ, Glidden DV, Jin C, Way LW, Patti MG. Has recognition of the relationship between mortality rates and hospital volume for major cancer surgery in California made a difference?: a follow-up analysis of another decade. Ann Surg. 2009;250(3):472–83.
23. Teh SH, Diggs BS, Deveney CW, Sheppard BC. Patient and hospital characteristics on the variance of perioperative outcomes for pancreatic resection in the United States: a plea for outcome-based and not volume-based referral guidelines. Arch Surg. 2009;144:713–21.
24. David JM, Kim S, Placencio-Hickok VR, Torosian A, Hendifar A, Tuli R. Adv Radiat Oncol. 2018;4(2):302–13.
25. Sargent D, Grothey A, Gray R. Time to initiation of adjuvant chemotherapy and survival in colorectal cancer. JAMA. 2011;306(11):1199.
26. Shapiro M, Chen Q, Huang Q, Boosalis VA, Yoon CH, Saund MS, Whang EE, Gold JS. Associations of socioeconomic variables with resection, stage, and survival in patients with early-stage pancreatic cancer. JAMA Surg. 2016;151(4):338–45.

27. Shah A, Chao KS, Ostbye T, Castleberry AW, Pietrobon R, Gloor B, Clary BM, White RR, Worni M. Trends in racial disparities in pancreatic cancer surgery. J Gastrointest Surg. 2013;17(11):1897–906.
28. Bos AC, van Erning FN, van Gestel YR, Creemers GJ, Punt CJ, van Oijen MG, Lemmens VE. Timing of adjuvant chemotherapy and its relation to survival among patients with stage III colon cancer. Eur J Cancer. 2015;51(17):2553–61.
29. Standeven L, Price Hiller J, Mulder K, Zhu G, Ghosh S, Spratlin JL. Impact of a dedicated cancer center surveillance program on guideline adherence for patients with stage II and III colorectal cancer. Clin Colorectal Cancer. 2013;12(2):103–12.
30. Hassan C, Kaminski MF, Repici A. How to ensure patient adherence to colorectal cancer screening and surveillance in your practice. Gastroenterology. 2018;155(2):252–7.
31. Levinson W, Lesser CS, Epstein RM. Developing physician communication skills for patient-centered care. Health Aff. 2010;29(7):1310–8.
32. Bredart A, Bouleuc C, Dolbeault S. Doctor-patient communication and satisfaction with care in oncology. Curr Opin Oncol. 2005;17(4):351–4.
33. Nestel D, Cooper S, Bryant M, Higgins V, Tabak D, Murtagh G, et al. Communication challenges in surgical oncology. Surg Oncol. 2011;20(3):155–61.

Human Factors Research in Orthopaedic Surgery

17

Mark Vrahas

Case Study

A 79-year-old female developed septic shock from a urinary tract infection that required multiple vasopressors to support her blood pressure. Her course was complicated by bilateral foot ischemia that would require below-the-knee amputations. The orthopaedic surgery team was consulted, and the plan was made to amputate the right foot. Since the patient was sedated and intubated, her husband consented to the right below-knee amputation. During morning rounds on the day of surgery, a resident thought the plan was to amputate both legs, so he wrote a big 'yes' on each thigh. Later in preoperative area, the attending marked the patient's right calf with a big yes without noticing the yes that was higher up. When the patient was rolled to the operating room (OR) and transferred to the operating room table, the circulating nurse saw that the left thigh was marked, and so he prepped the left leg rather than the right. When the attending entered the room, he noted the prepped leg and scrubbed in preparation for the amputation. A timeout was conducted, which stated that the right below-the-knee amputation was going to occur, and the attending stopped the case. A huddle was conducted to determine the correct procedure. The patient was prepped again for a right below-the-knee amputation and the case was reported for review.

Overview

The move towards value-based payments has prompted recent interest in human factors research in general and orthopaedic surgery. Value is defined as quality/costs and addressing both the numerator and denominator is critical for success in the

M. Vrahas (✉)
Orthopaedics, Cedars-Sinai Medical Center, Los Angeles, CA, USA
e-mail: mark.vrahas@cshs.org

T. N. Cohen et al. (eds.), *Human Factors in Surgery*,
https://doi.org/10.1007/978-3-030-53127-0_17

developing paradigm. The operating rooms account for up to 40% of hospital costs and generate 70% of hospital revenues [1]. Thus, improving operating room efficiency is critical to hospitals' financial stability. At the same time, indiscriminately reducing resources to save money can affect quality. Improving value for orthopaedic procedures is particularly important since Medicare expenditures for total joint arthroplasty are substantial and Centers for Medicare & Medicaid Services (CMS) has mandated bundled payments for total joints in many markets across the country. Consequently, the bulk of orthopaedic human factors research has focused on improving value in operating rooms either through improving quality by avoiding harm or decreasing costs by improving efficiency. Although there is a great deal of literature regarding operating room efficiency, in general, there is relatively little focusing on orthopaedics directly. This chapter will review the literature surrounding these efforts.

Safety

Even before the current interest in value, surgeries performed on the wrong site or on the wrong patient were recognized as a problem particularly in orthopaedic surgery. The problem was first documented in 1988 by the Medical Defense Union in the UK and, subsequently, in 1993, by the Canadian Medical Protective Association. The data prompted the Canadian Orthopaedic Association to review the problem and ultimately to adopt an initiative to 'Operate Through Your Initials' [2].

In 1997, the American Academy of Orthopaedic Surgeons (AAOS) organized a task force to examine the problem. Working with data from malpractice insurance providers, the task force estimated that the average orthopaedic surgeon had a 25% chance of preforming a wrong-site surgery at some point in his or her career. Based on their findings, the task force recommended a 'Sign Your Site' programme, and the AAOS adopted the recommendation in 1997 [3]. In 2000, the Institutes of Medicine report, *To Err Is Human*, drew attention to medical errors and generated even greater interest in preventing wrong-site surgeries. As a result, in 2004, the Joint Commission introduced the Universal Protocol and required its use for accreditation. The protocol standardized perioperative protocols for proper patient identification, surgical site marking and a timeout procedure prior to incision [4]. Despite these advances, there has been little research looking at this human factors problem [5].

The term wrong-site surgery literally refers to surgeries performed at the wrong anatomic location. However, the term is generally used to include surgeries performed on the wrong patient and incorrect procedures. The true incidence of wrong-site surgery is unknown and is likely much higher than official reports. The Joint Commission considers wrong-site surgery a sentinel event, but reporting is voluntary. From 2004 to 2013, a total of 1,037 wrong-site surgeries were reported to the joint commission. However, since reporting is voluntary, the Joint Commission believes this number underestimates the total [4]. The most accurate and complete data on wrong-site surgery come from the Pennsylvania Patient Authority. In 2004, the authority mandated the reporting of wrong-site events and has provided annual reports and analysis since that time. Since 2004, 731 cases were reported. A total of 59% of wrong-site procedures were procedures performed on the wrong side, with nerve blocks making up the bulk of these cases. Wrong anatomic site procedures made up 32% of the reported cases, and the wrong procedure was performed in 9% of the cases [5]. Overall, the number of wrong-site surgeries in Pennsylvania has decreased since 2004, but since the denominator is not known, it is difficult to know if this represents true improvement. There continues to be at least one wrong-site procedure reported each week in Pennsylvania [5]

Despite the intense interest in medical errors and wrong-site procedures, there is little evidence that we are making headway and almost no human factors research examining the problem. There is no scientific data demonstrating that universal protocols and sign your site initiatives decrease the rates of wrong-site surgery, and the numbers are hard to interpret. It is difficult to determine the true incidence, not only because of underreporting but also because the denominator of potential cases where wrong-site surgery might occur is difficult to determine. In addition, wrong-site surgeries are sufficiently rare to require huge number of accurately reported cases to show a statistically significant reduction in occurrence [6].

In 2007, Clarke et al. reviewed data collected by the Pennsylvania Safety Authority to determine factors contributing to wrong-site surgeries. Wrong-site surgeries were divided into four categories: (1) errors not reaching the patient, (2) errors reaching the patient but not violating the informed consent, (3) initiated but aborted procedures and (4) completed wrong-site procedures. They identified 427 reports of wrong-site surgery in the PA_PSR database over a 30-month period. Overall, 239 cases were reported as near misses, and errors were corrected prior to procedure initiation. Of the 188 cases that got past the initial screening procedures, 30% were corrected after initial imaging studies, 18% were corrected after the procedure had started and 44% were never corrected. Based on their analysis, they suggested that a single timeout just prior to surgery inadequately guarded against wrong-site surgeries. In their series, 21 wrong-site procedures occurred despite adequate timeout processes, and 12 of these resulted in completed wrong-site procedures. Similarly, preoperative marking was not always effective as 17 incorrect markings were corrected with an extensive verification process prior to surgery. In 10 cases, markings did prevent wrong site errors, but accurate site marking failed to prevent wrong-site procedures in 16 cases, and in 6 cases, correct marks were not noticed until after the procedure was completed [6]. They also noted that patients often misidentified the surgical site. Moreover, they suggest that preventing wrong-site surgery requires verification at multiple steps in the process, beginning with accurate information from the surgeon's office that accompanies the patient and can be reviewed at each step in the process. Ultimately, the surgeon must be engaged in the process [6].

There has been much recent interest in checklists to improve safety and efficiency. Again, however, there has been little work specific to orthopaedic procedures. Surgical checklists are designed to reinforce accepted safety procedures to minimize human error in busy operating rooms. In addition, they are thought to facilitate communication, enabling all members of the team to speak up when something is amiss. The World Health Organization (WHO) Surgical Safety Checklist is a high-level example and is meant to address safety at three distinct stages: 'sign in' (before anaesthesia), 'time out' (before incision) and 'sign out' (at completion). In 2004, the Joint Commission on Accreditation of Healthcare Organizations enacted The Universal Protocol with a 'timeout' prior to incision and a standard checklist to ensure the timeout covered the appropriate material [7].

The Safe Surgery Saves Lives Study Group evaluated a 19-item surgical safety checklist based on the WHO's Guidelines for Safe Surgery. The study included eight hospitals from around the world. The hospitals and patient populations were diverse, representing both developed and developing nations. Overall, there was a significant drop in inpatient complications from 11% to 7%, which they attributed to the introduction of the checklist. Although the evidence for improvement was robust, the mechanism for this improvement was less clear. The checklists were not consistently effective. Before the introduction of checklists, the six safety elements evaluated were preformed 34% of the time. After the safety list introduction, the six elements were performed 56% of the time. Multiple factors, including the Hawthorne effect, may have contributed to the improved outcomes. Nevertheless, checklists did increase adherence to appropriate preoperative antibiotic administration from 56% to 88% and could easily explain a decrease in post-operative infections [8]. In a more rigorous study of checklists, Haugen et al. found that the introduction of surgical checklists substantially improved adherence to best practices. In a study of 3,702 procedures, including a substantial volume of orthopaedic procedures, they found that high-quality implementation of checklists significantly improved warming blanket use and the appropriate use of antibiotics, and could have contributed to a decrease in infections and blood transfusions to these process improvements [9]. Moreover, it does appear that surgical checklists can improve outcomes by improving processes. Nevertheless, for checklists to be effective, it is essential that they are taken seriously and are more than a written task [7].

Operating Room Efficiency

There has been a great deal of interest in improving OR efficiency. [1] Part of this effort has included an interest in applying quality improvement methodologies developed and proven successful in other industries to healthcare [1]. Nicolay et al. conducted a systemic review to elucidate the use of these methodologies in healthcare. For this review, they identified only 34 empirical studies in the peer-reviewed literature that evaluated hospital-based surgical patients, described a named quality improvement methodology and had appropriate statistical methods. There was only one randomized controlled trial and, unfortunately, no studies evaluating orthopaedic procedures. There were nine Continuous Quality Improvement studies, five Six Sigma, five Total Quality Management, five Statistical Process Control or Statistical Quality Control, five plan-do-check-act or plan-do-study-act, and one Lean Six Sigma. In general, the review suggested that these methodologies can be used to reduce infection rates and improve operating room efficiency. However, the data quality was suboptimal. Time periods covered by the studies were variable, and most described continuous improvement efforts not accounting for the multiple other changes that might have occurred during the study periods. In most cases, the positive results could have resulted from a Hawthorne effect, with improvements resulting simply by engaging staff. Moreover, there is room for more rigorous evaluation of these methodologies, especially in orthopaedic surgery [10].

Even though the literature has not been extensive, orthopaedic procedures are an important profit driver for hospitals and consequently have received some attention. The demand for hip and knee arthroplasties has been increasing, but reimbursements have been decreasing, thus driving the need for increased efficiency to maintain margins [11]. Addressing OR efficiency is a true human factors problem, but a complex one. In a project to improve OR efficiency for arthroplasty cases, Attarian et al. improved on-time starts from 60% to 90% and turnovers from greater than 60 minutes to 35 minutes. Process analysis prior to intervention identified multiple human factors leading to inefficiencies. Patient, nurse, surgeon, anaesthesiologist and support staff factors, as well as process difficulties and instruments issues, all contributed to the problems [11].

The common characteristics among successful OR efficiency improvement projects are high-level institutional support, careful and extensive analysis of existing processes, and involvement and buy-in from all stake holders. These three factors are interdependent. The institution must commit to the effort and provide the extensive resources necessary for analysis and project management. Busy clinicians and clinical staff cannot be expected to provide the in-depth analysis necessary for success and do not have the time or background to manage the project. Extensive analysis usually demonstrates that the problems are multifactorial, and addressing one component of the problem is rarely successful. Finally, providing stakeholders with the in-depth analysis eliminates the common perception that one part of the team is to blame and allows all stakeholders to work together towards a common goal.

The successful project described earlier begins with a detailed analysis to understand the starting point [11]. This required an interdisciplinary assessment team of surgeons, anaesthesiologists, OR nurses, support personnel, sterile processing, post-anaesthesia and intermediate care, and hospital administrators. The project was led by hospital personnel trained in Six Sigma techniques. They conducted extensive real-time analysis of patient flow and OR processes, developed process flow maps and presented the data to the multidisciplinary efficiency team. Only then, with the engagement of all stakeholders, did they begin to design strategies to address the multiple issues [11]. A successful effort at the Mayo Clinic followed a similar model. The first step in the project was to develop detailed process flow maps and to engage a multidisciplinary team [12]. These efforts require a great deal of time and are resource intensive, but they are critical to success. Einstein said, 'If I had only one hour to save the world, I would spend fifty-five minutes defining the problem, and only five minutes finding the solution' [13].

The Mayo Clinic in Florida took a different approach to improving OR efficiency. Most OR efficiency projects have worked to increase throughput by eliminating waste and improving processes. The Mayo Clinic addressed the problem by managing the flow of surgical patients into hospital and operating rooms. Other industries predict demand and optimally manage flow to provide consistent service. These efforts depend on understanding and managing variability. To address the problem of flow, they did an extensive analysis of emergent, urgent, semi-urgent and elective cases to understand variability. They created mathematical models to predict flow with various scenarios and picked the best. They then rearranged surgeon block time and case type to optimize flow. It is important to note that these changes were made without regard to surgeon schedules or preferences. All changes were made to optimize flow. They were successful from the hospital's perspective. Surgical volume increased 4%, overtime staffing decreased 27%, same-day schedule changes decreased 70% and net operating margin improved 28%. Despite this success, the authors note a critical consideration. A huge culture shift was necessary to implement this model. Typically, hospitals schedule cases to accommodate the surgeon. The Mayo model forced surgeons to compromise for the financial benefit of the hospital. During implementation, the resulting tension between the hospital and the surgeons became intense, and it is easy to image how similar efforts could destroy moral and drive surgeons away [14]. Moreover, culture is a human factors component that should not be underestimated. There are aspects of surgical culture in general that make process improvement projects difficult, and each institution has cultural aspects that make cookie-cutter solutions impossible.

Resident Training

Another human factors problem to consider is our traditional model for resident education. Pugely et al. studied the effect of resident participation on 66,817 orthopaedic cases using the American College of Surgeons National Surgical Quality Improvement Program data set. They studied six orthopaedic procedural domains, including total joint arthroplasties, revision total joint arthroplasties, advanced arthroscopies, lower extremity traumas and spine arthrodesis. Although resident involvement did not increase mortality, it did increase the odds of complication for revision total joint arthroplasty, lower extremity trauma and spine arthrodesis. Operative time was greater with resident involvement in all procedural domains [15]. There is some hope that surgical simulation will mitigate this problem, but there is limited evidence that this is the case. Frank et al. reported a systemic review of arthroscopic training models, finding 19 articles meeting inclusion criteria. A total of 12 articles examined experience levels with simulator performance, and all found a positive correlation. Six studies found improvement after training. A single study commented on operating room performance [16]. Howells et al. evaluated the effectiveness of simulator training on the ability of surgical trainees to perform diagnostic arthroscopy of the knee. Twenty junior residents were randomized to either receive simulator training or not, and their performance in the OR was evaluated by blinded consultants. The simulator-trained group performed significantly better than the untrained group. (17) Moreover, as noted above, the negative consequences of resident involvement occurred with open procedures, not arthroscopy, and there is no literature evaluating the effectiveness of simulator training for open orthopaedic procedures [15].

In summary, there is little human factors research specific to orthopaedics. Most studies are related to OR efficiency and safety, but, most often, orthopaedic procedures are included in a general analysis of OR process for all procedures. Hopefully, the importance and prevalence of orthopaedic procedures will stimulate further research. Wrong-site surgery remains a major concern in orthopaedics, and continued research is necessary to mitigate this problem. Orthopaedic procedures, especially knee and hip arthroplasty, are important hospital profit centres, but with decreasing reimbursements, improvements in the human factors problem of OR efficiency is critical for the financial health of our hospitals. Finally, human factors research into safer and more effective ways to train our residents is essential.

Lessons Learnt

- The average orthopaedic surgeon has a significant chance of preforming a wrong-site surgery at some point in his or her career.
- Preventing wrong-site surgery requires verification at multiple steps in the process, beginning with accurate information that can be reviewed at each step, as well as an engaged surgeon,
- Characteristics among successful OR efficiency improvement projects are high-level institutional support, careful and extensive analysis of existing processes, and involvement and buy-in from all stake holders.

References

1. Healey T, El-Othmani M, Healey J, Peterson T, Saleh K. Improving operating room efficiency, part 1: general managerial and preoperative strategies. JBJS Rev. 2015;3(10):30.
2. Terry CS. Wrong-site surgery-a preventable complication. Clin Orthop Relat Res. 2005;Number 433:26–9.
3. Wong D, Herndon J, Canale T. An AOA critical issue. Medical errors in orthopaedics: practical pointers for prevention. J Bone Joint Surg Am. 2002;84(11):2097–100.
4. Santiesteban L, Hutzler L, Bosco JA, Robb W. Wrong-site surgery in orthopaedics: prevalence, risk factors, and strategies for prevention. JBJS Rev. 2016;4(1):01874474-201601000-00003.
5. Clark JR, Johnston J, Finley ED. Getting surgery right. Ann Surg. 2007;246(3):395–403.
6. Haugen AS, Sevdalis N, Softeland E. Impact of the World Health Organization surgical safety checklist on patient safety. Anesthesiology. 2019;131(2):420–5.
7. Haynes AB, Weiser TG, Berry WR, Lipsitz SR, Breizat AH, Dellinger EP, Herbosa T, Joseph S, Kibatala PL, Lapitan MC, Merry AF, Moorthy K, Reznick RK, Taylor B, Gawande AA. Safe Surgery Saves Lives Study Group. A surgical safety checklist to reduce morbidity and mortality in a global population. N Engl J Med. 2009;360(5):491–9.
8. Haugen AS, Waehle HV, Almeland SK, Harthug S, Sevdalis N, Eide GE, Nortvedt MW, Smith I, Softeland E. Causal analysis of World Health Organization's surgical checklist implementation quality and impact on care processes and patient outcomes: secondary analysis from a large stepped wedge cluster randomized controlled trail in Norway. Ann Surg. 2019;269(2):283–90.

9. Nicolay CR, Purkayastha S, Greenhalgh A, Benn J, Chaturvedi S, Phillips N, Darzi A. Systematic review of the application of quality improvement methodologies from the manufacturing industry to surgical healthcare. Br J Surg. 2012;99(3):324–35.
10. Attarian DE, Wahl JE, Wellman SS, Bolognesi MP. Developing a high-efficiency operating room for total joint arthroplasty in an academic setting. Clin Orthop Relat Res. 2013;471(6):1832–6.
11. Cima RR, Brown MJ, Hebl JR, Moore R, Rogers JC, Kollengode A, Amstutz GJ, Wesibrod CA, Narr BJ, Deschamps C. Surgical process improvement tream, Mayo Clinic, Rochester. J Am Coll Surg. 2011;213(1):83–92.
12. "If I had only one hour to save the world, I would spend fifty-five minutes defining the problem, and only five minutes finding the solution." Albert Einstein.
13. Smith CD, Spackman T, Brommer K, Stewart MW, Vizzini M, Frye J, Rupp WC. Re-engineering the operating room using the variability methodology to improve health care value. J Am Coll Surg. 2013;216(4):559–68.
14. Pugely AJ, Gao Y, Martin CT, Callagh JJ, Weinstein SL, March JL. The effect of resident participation on short-term outcomes after orthopaedic surgery. Clin Orthop Relat Res. 2014;472(7):2290–300.
15. Frank RM, Erickson B, Frank JM, Bush-Joseph CA, Bach BR Jr, Cole BJ, Romeo AA, Provencher MT, Verma NN. Utility of modern arthroscopic stimulator training models. Arthroscopy. 2014;30(1):121–33.
16. Howells NR, Gill HS, Carr AJ, Price AJ, Rees JL. Transferring simulated arthroscopic skills to the operating theatre: a randomized blinded study. J Bone Joint Surg Br. 2008;90(4):494–9.

18 Human Factors in Pediatric Surgery

David Bliss

Case Study

A 12-year-old male sustained a crush injury to his lower limb due to a strike by a motor vehicle at a high rate of speed that pinned him against a fixed object. After a short response time from the Emergency Medical Services (EMS), with an unknown amount of blood loss at the scene, he was taken to the nearest trauma center. At the initial institution, he was determined to have an isolated injury to the proximal lower leg with diminished pulses but intact sensation and movement in the ipsilateral foot. Studies from the initial institution included a hemoglobin level of 14 g/dL; plane films demonstrating a comminuted, open, posteriorly displaced proximal tibia and fibula fractures; and a computed tomography (CT) angiogram revealing extravasation of contrast at the infrapopliteal arterial trifurcation with two-vessel runoff. His vital signs and cognition were recorded as normal prior to transfer to the second institution.

Information for transfer was transmitted via the receiving institution's communication center and included the mechanism of injury and the clinical, laboratory, and radiographic findings at the referring center. Initial EMS documentation was not provided in the materials accompanying the patient in transfer. Transport was executed by the receiving hospitals team, consisting of pediatric transport nurses.

At the receiving institution, a level 2 trauma activation was initiated based upon a preexisting protocol for transfers from other trauma centers, independent of mechanism of injury. The patient was met by a senior surgical trainee, emergency department trainees and attending physician, and trauma team nurses and technicians. The child was documented to have an isolated injury on physical exam and normal vital signs for age. A repeat hemoglobin revealed a lower value of 10.6 g/dL. No coagulation studies, type and screen or type and cross, or other salient laboratory or radiographic tests were obtained. After review of the plain films, an orthopedic consult

D. Bliss (✉)
Pediatric Surgery, Cedars-Sinai Medical Center, Los Angeles, CA, USA
e-mail: David.Bliss@cshs.org

T. N. Cohen et al. (eds.), *Human Factors in Surgery*,
https://doi.org/10.1007/978-3-030-53127-0_18

was obtained, and the orthopedic team elected to take the child to the operating room. The attending trauma surgeon was not informed of the plan to proceed immediately to the operating room, and the supervising trainee was neither aware of the contrast extravasation demonstrated on CT angiography nor the change in serum hemoglobin. Intravenous fluids were administered at maintenance rate and appropriate antibiotics were given.

The attending pediatric anesthesiologist was informed that the child had a complex, open bony repair in need of urgent repair, but that the child was "hemodynamically stable." The finding of the hemoglobin level at the receiving institution and plain films were relayed to the anesthesiologist, but prior laboratory findings as well as the results of the CT angiography were not discussed. At the time of induction of anesthesia, the care team included the attending and resident anesthesiologists, circulating nurse and technician, and the orthopedic team. There was no evidence of ongoing external blood loss.

Upon induction of anesthesia, the child became profoundly hypotensive. The anesthesiologist responded with intravenous epinephrine, recheck of the serum hemoglobin (7 g/dL), directing a call to the blood bank to obtain type-specific blood, perform a chest radiograph (normal), and a call to the pediatric intensivist to perform a focused abdominal sonography for trauma (normal). After a successful hemodynamic resuscitation and determination that there were no other foci of blood loss, a vascular surgeon and the orthopedic surgeon jointly completed definitive vascular repair and fixation of the bony injuries with return of normal distal blood flow. The patient had an uneventful postoperative course.

Analysis

Identifiable Human Factors Issues

Manifestly, this case illustrates errors of communication, judgment, resource allocation, and preparation that combined in what Reason has labeled a "swiss cheese" model. Taken temporally, these may be characterized as follows:

1. *Information relay between institutions and clinicians*: While the discussion between providers in a transfer phone call should, ideally, relay all relevant clinical information, set context, and establish priority, it is clear that this did not occur. Despite an attempt to provide the correct data, the receiving clinician appears not to have noted or prioritized the finding of a normal initial serum hemoglobin and the angiographic findings of contrast extravasation. Furthermore, the lack of EMS paperwork may have contributed to a lack of understanding of the severity of injury. The serial transmission of information from EMS to initial trauma surgeon followed by interpretation from the referring to the receiving surgeon apparently failed to communicate the energy transfer, total time from injury, and external blood loss at the scene.
2. *Trainee experience and judgment*: The senior resident who accepted the patient transfer appears to not have registered the significance or, perhaps, presence of

the vascular injury. As a consequence, the individual was presumably inattentive to the findings of diminished distal pulse quality on examination as well as the 4 g/dL drop in serum hemoglobin between the two institutions. This gap led the trainee to believe that this was an "isolated orthopedic injury," which did not warrant either notification of the trauma attending or trauma team participation in the operative procedure.

3. *Secondary and tertiary communications*: Having determined that the injury only required orthopedic intervention, the trainee relayed truncated information to both the supervising trainee and the attending anesthesiologist. Neither of these individuals inquired as to whether the hemoglobin level had changed, was cross-matched blood available, and was there any consideration of vascular injury. In addition, no conversations were held to explicitly transmit how the central nervous system (CNS), spine, and abdomen had been evaluated.
4. *Preparation*: Though the patient was known to be headed for a complex surgical procedure in the early morning hours, numerous potential risks that could have been constrained were unrecognized by all parties. First, failure to communicate to the most senior trauma clinician eliminated the option for timely input of the most experienced, responsible individual. Second, explicit clearance of other major body areas as potential sources of bleeding would have eliminated the delays and confusion when the patient's physiology unexpectedly deteriorated in the operating room. The clinicians extended an institutional policy regarding screening methods for abdominal injury in children who are *not* undergoing operation but who may have serial examinations to the current circumstance. However, the inability to re-examine the abdomen and the lack of reliable preoperative imaging created a void in knowledge that contributed to confusion and delay. Third, failure to organize appropriate blood products for a significant injury with large potential for blood loss led to additional delays and substitution of less optimal therapies. Fourth, failure to recognize the need for an attending surgeon with vascular experience and the value of trauma team participation in emergency trauma operations was a judgment error.
5. *Explicit emergency communication protocols*: In the absence of an explicit protocol for communication of a substantive change in patient status, the anesthesiologist had to direct communications to multiple departments while continuing to manage the patient. Had a trauma team member been present, either by policy or as a behavioral norm, he or she would have assumed responsibility for these matters. In the absence of their presence, explicit communication to the operating room team of a responsible trauma team member to contact in the event of such a change would have also streamlined care, eliminated confusion over data, and expedited marshalling of resources.

Background

Though human factors have been extensively researched in medicine and, more recently, in surgery, there is a dearth of information in pediatric surgery. To a significant degree, this reflects both the nature of pediatric care as well as its relatively small share of the medical cost structure. Indeed, similar disparities may be found between adult and pediatric research with respect to pharmacology and other therapeutics, randomized clinical trials, and value-based comparative studies. The vast majority of pediatric disciplines frequently rely upon off-label approaches such as the application of medicines tested only in adults, clinician experience and opinion, and small studies. Moreover, surgical safety systems, such as operative "time-outs," have largely been developed within Adult care and their effectiveness within pediatric surgical disciplines have not been studied adequately.

Despite the paucity of data and experience with human factors research in children, there is reason to believe that this will have similar impacts. Avoidable adverse clinical events are increasingly recognized to be due to one of several factors: (1) variability of human biological response; (2) limitations of current knowledge and science; and (3) human errors. While the impacts may be more evident and even severe in adults due to comorbidities, complexity of illness, and large numbers of patients, it is likely that the cognitive errors, systems failures, and group dynamics that are at play in adults also affect children.

Heuristics

A heuristic approach to clinical care employs the commonly used practical method not guaranteed to be optimal or perfect, but sufficient for the immediate goals. In a thorough review of human cognitive processing, "Thinking Fast and Slow," Nobel Laureate Daniel Kahneman describes the automaticity of human behavior [1]. In particular, he focuses on heuristics, algorithmic responses to circumstances of uncertainty, which may be adaptive or maladaptive. Examples include anchoring, availability, substitution, optimism and loss aversion, framing, sunk cost, and overconfidence. He notes a long history of psychology research, demonstrating that educated persons are no less subject to these cognitive errors and, in the specific case of physicians, may be more likely to demonstrate overconfidence and underestimate the role of chance. Though not addressed in Kahneman's work, it is reasonable to assume that surgeons caring for children are no less likely to manifest these limitations. Indeed, it may well be that the relative void of high-value scientific data in the field may well be filled by heuristics and assumptions with potentially deleterious effects.

However, action under circumstances of uncertainty is a necessary component of pediatric care in particular. Many patients are unable to communicate at all, while others lack the cognitive or communication skills to inform clinicians' decision-making. The "adaptability" of clinicians in such circumstances may be protective against error [2]. Indeed, Reason has labeled this function as "requisite imagination," wherein individuals may employ prior knowledge, experience, and observations to reach reasonable conclusions [3]. These authors go on to suggest that a temporospatial community of clinician knowledge (physician, nursing, technician) is potentially protective. Certainly, the prevailing belief among clinicians has generally been that the "wisdom of experience" combined with the intellectual and social controls of the clinician community should be optimal. Manifestly, however, error rates associated with human factors issues remain excessive. Based on the work of Kahneman and other research psychologists, pediatric care and medicine, in general, may need to revisit other means to address human factors beyond bolstering traditional views of the value of individual or collective clinician judgment.

Associated Disciplines

Pediatric Anesthesia

It is impossible to address matters of pediatric surgical care and human factors without an examination of the role of pediatric anesthesia. Though this is a discipline that has existed as a de facto sub-specialty for decades, it was only recently granted specialty certification by the American Board of Anesthesia. In addition, highly specialized training has emerged for congenital heart surgery, regional/pain, and others. Nevertheless, sub-specialty Board certification is sufficiently new that the majority of pediatric anesthesia providers, both physician and nurse anesthetist, do not have accredited fellowship training in the discipline.

The diverse type of providers, their training and experience, and the resources that are available to promote safety are highly variable. In a study from Birmingham, England, researchers retrospectively examined adverse anesthetic events in the pediatric operating room of a major children's hospital. Human factors were determined to have contributed to 42.5% of events including, "errors in judgment 43%, failure to check 17.8%, technical failures of skill 9.2%, inexperience 7.7%, inattention/distraction 5.6% and communication issues 5.6%" [4]. The authors' findings suggest ample opportunity for improvement of pediatric surgical care through the improvement of human factors in anesthesia services.

Pediatric Intensive Care

Critically ill pediatric surgical patients are frequently cared for by a combined team of intensive care and surgical clinicians. In a study from Great Britain, researchers noted that children were more than twice as likely to suffer adverse impacts from a medication error as adults [5]. The pediatric ICU environment suffers from a medication error rate between 11% and 18% [6, 7]. A recent study using Hierarchical Task Analysis and practitioner interviews based upon Reason's "Swiss Cheese" model recognized 30 sub-tasks that are essential to safe prescribing [8]. The researchers identified cognitive stress, distraction, fatigue, time pressure, perceived low value of diligence, lack of pediatric-specific pharmacological information, disregard for protocols and guidelines, and hierarchy as significant human factors.

Reason described three types of organizational control processes to promote safe systems performance in high-risk environments—administrative rules, policies and procedures, social norms, and self (a personal understanding of what is safe and what is not) [7]. However, Sutherland et al. observed that "administrative controls are poorly designed and inaccessible, and lacking information to support knowledge-based behaviours. Thus, only social controls are available to mitigate prescribing errors…" [3] Strategies to mitigate fatigue, promote task focus and minimize distractions, automate safety checks, and build sub-task articulation and simplification may have value across many pediatric clinical domains.

Pediatric Surgical Disciplines

Congenital Heart Surgery

Perhaps the best-studied domain with respect to human factors is congenital cardiac surgery. Indeed, Dr. Reason's early work included the observation of 243 arterial switch procedures in Great Britain [9]. Perhaps not surprisingly, the number of serious intraoperative events correlated with outcome despite 90% being addressed ("compensated") at the time of their occurrence. Innumerable studies have also demonstrated that team volume and structure of care delivery impact outcomes [10, 11]. Follow-on work has suggested that there is currently an asymptote for adverse intraoperative events, independent of the severity of the cardiac lesion. These appear to have limited impacts if a team is well trained in recognition and compensation [12]. Using a rigorous real-time, intraoperative evaluation tool, the team at Boston Children's Hospital demonstrated that technical skill has been identified as a critical human factor in congenital heart surgery outcomes [13]. Procedures that received low technical scores resulted in longer hospital stays, more days on mechanical ventilation and in the ICU, and increased complication rates. Case morbidity was associated with the technical score, irrespective of case complexity [14].

Notably, the congenital heart surgery literature has recognized transitions of care and communication as a substantial contributor to error. In one interventional study, researchers found that a rigorous information transfer methodology reduced technical errors from 6.24 to 1.52 and critical omissions from 6.33 to 2.38 per patient handover [15]. Though a thorough discussion of the implications of these and other findings is beyond the scope of this chapter, the research suggests that human factors such as skill, experience, cognition, and team dynamics have significant impacts on the outcomes of complex congenital heart lesions.

Pediatric General Surgery

In the past decade, there has been an increasing recognition among pediatric general surgeons for the need to promote safety. In a recent survey of North American surgeons regarding safety culture, surgeons in academic practices or leadership positions were more likely to be actively engaged in safety practices and to feel comfortable with their own children undergoing procedures in their institution as compared to those in private practice [16]. Drawing from the experience of trauma systems, the American Pediatric Surgical Association has developed a comprehensive set of standards for pediatric surgical care in North America [17]. In this publication, the consortium detailed published data demonstrating the value of specialized centers, particularly for the care of surgical neonates, intensive care, injured adolescents and children, and congenital heart disease. In addition, the authors strongly supported the need for "appropriate pediatric anesthesia expertise," dedicated perioperative care spaces staffed by specialized team members, and personnel trained in age-specific emergency resuscitation. Additional clinician expertise in radiology, general pediatrics, and emergency room is recommended to optimize care delivery. Strictly speaking, the referenced document does not directly evaluate the impact of human factors on outcomes in pediatric surgical care. However, the underpinning data suggest that limiting complex pediatric surgical care to centers with clinician training, experience, and skill is generally associated with better outcomes.

Further directed research is needed to determine the breadth and depth of human factors impacts on pediatric surgical care. To date, limitations have included the relative dearth of objective standards, extension of adult principles without verification of their applicability in neonates, children, and adolescents, and the small numbers and diverse case types that limit data power.

Conclusion

Pediatric surgery is in the early stages of recognizing the impacts of human factors on clinical quality, safety, and outcomes. Data and experience, including the vignette provided, suggest that there are ample opportunities to improve skill, training, experience, judgment, communication, preparation, culture/norms, and use of policies and procedures within this discipline. While some of these matters are undergoing change at a rapid pace, including surgical safety checklists, time-outs, and improvement in handoffs, many others have yet to be addressed.

Key Points

- Pediatric surgery is increasingly recognizing the impacts of human factors on clinical quality, safety, and outcomes.
- While pediatric surgery has implemented human factors interventions such as surgical safety checklists, time-outs, and improvement in handoffs, many others are yet to be addressed.
- Pediatric surgery requires adaptability as many children are unable to communicate, while others lack the cognitive or communication skills to inform clinicians' decision-making.
- A heuristic approach may employ practical methods sufficient for immediate goals but could also lead to systemic errors.

References

1. Kahneman D. Thinking fast and slow. Farrar, Straus and Giroux, 2011. ISBN978-0374275631.
2. Hollnagel E, Braithwaite J, Wears RL. Resilient health care: volume 2 : the resilience of everyday clinical work. 2015.
3. Reason J, Parker D, Lawton R. Organizational controls and safety: the varieties of rule-related behaviour. J Occup Organ Psychol. 1998;71:289–304. https://doi.org/10.1111/j.2044-8325.1998.tb00678.x.
4. Marcus R. Human factors in pediatric anesthesia incidents. Pediatr Anesth. 2005; https://doi.org/10.1111/j.1460-9592.2005.01771.x.
5. Department of Health. National service framework for children, young people and maternity services: medicines for children and young people. London; 2007.
6. Cimino MA, Kirschbaum MS, Brodsky L, et al. Assessing medication prescribing errors in pediatric intensive care units. Pediatr Crit Care Med. 2004;5:124–32. https://doi.org/10.1097/01.PCC.0000112371.26138.E8.
7. Sutherland A, Talken-Sinclair J, Barber R. Reducing prescribing errors in a British PICU. Pediatr Crit Care Med. 2011;12:A148.
8. Sutherland A, Ashcroft DM, Phipps DL. Exploring the human factors of prescribing errors in paediatric intensive care units. Arch Dis Child. 2019;104:588–95.
9. Carthey J, de Leval MR, Reason JT. The human factor in cardiac surgery: errors and near misses in a high technology medical domain. Ann Thorac Surg. 2001;72:300–5.
10. Bacha EA. Patient safety and human factors in pediatric cardiac surgery. Pediatr Cardiol. 2007;28:116. https://doi.org/10.1007/s00246-006-1448-3.
11. Hannan EL, Racz M, Kavey R, Quaegebeur JM, Williams R. Pediatric cardiac surgery: the effect of hospital and surgeon volume on in-hospital mortality. Pediatrics. 1998;101:963–9.
12. Galvan C, Bacha EA, Mohr JJ, Starr JP, Barach P. The role of human factors in patient safety during pediatric cardiac surgery. Anesthesiology. 2004;101:A1264.
13. Larrazabal LA, del Nido PJ, Jenkins KJ, Gauvreau K, Lacro R, Colan SD, et al. Measurement of technical performance in surgery for congenital heart disease: a pilot study. Ann Thorac Surg. 2007;83:179–84.
14. Nathan M, Karamichalis JM, Liu H, Gauvreau K, Colan S, Saia M, Pigula F-TF, Emani S, Biard C, Mayer JE, del Nido PJ. Technical performance scores are strongly associated with early mortality, postoperative adverse events, and intensive care unit length of stay-analysis of consecutive discharges for two years. J Thorac Cardiovasc Surg. 2014;147:389–96.
15. Joy BF, Elliott E, Hardy C, Sullivan C, Backer CL, Kane JM. Standardized multidisciplinary protocol improves handover of cardiac surgery patients to the intensive care unit. Pediatr Crit Care Med. 2011;12(3):304–8.
16. Berman L, Rangel S, Goldin A, Skarda D, Ottosen M, Bliss D, Valusek P, Fallat M, Tsao K, APSA Quality and Safety Committee. Safety culture among pediatric surgeons: a national survey of attitudes and perceptions of patient safety. J Pediatr Surg. 2018;53(3):381–95. https://doi.org/10.1016/j.jpedsurg.2017.09.011. Epub 2017 Oct 6. PMID: 29111082
17. Oldham KT. Optimal resources for children's surgical care. J Am Coll Surg. 2014;218(3):479.

Plastic and Reconstructive Surgery

19

Edward Ray, Dhivya R. Srinivasa, and Randy Sherman

What Is Reconstructive Surgery?

Reconstructive surgery involves the repair and replacement of missing tissues as well as the improvement of function following trauma, cancer surgery, or in cases of congenital deformity. Tissues may be relocated from distant parts of the body or may be locally rearranged to repair defects. Reconstructive surgeons commonly work in close coordination with other surgical subspecialties, restoring physical integrity after a variety of antecedent procedures. Accordingly, clear communication, anticipation, and planning are critical for an optimal outcome.

Case Study

An example is provided to illustrate the importance of communication, planning, and anticipation in optimizing outcomes and the efficiency of the reconstructive surgical team.

The cancer surgeon is planning to remove a recurrent squamous cell cancer of the mouth that is invading the left side of the mandible. The patient is a VIP who has just arrived in the clinic from out-of-town, referred by a respected colleague. The cancer surgeon would like to perform the surgery as soon as possible and clears his schedule for the following day to accommodate the patient. He recruits his plastic surgery colleague to perform the reconstruction. An outside PET-CT scan has been performed and shows possible metastasis to the neck lymph nodes, so a radical left neck dissection is also planned. The cancer surgeon explains that in addition to a tracheostomy and neck dissection, he will be removing a portion of the left mandible and would like to have the oral floor and mandible reconstructed. The plastic

E. Ray (✉) · D. R. Srinivasa · R. Sherman
Department of Surgery, Cedars-Sinai Medical Center, Los Angeles, CA, USA
e-mail: Edward.Ray@cshs.org

T. N. Cohen et al. (eds.), *Human Factors in Surgery*,
https://doi.org/10.1007/978-3-030-53127-0_19

surgeon prefers to have lower extremity imaging and 3D models made to plan reconstruction, but there is insufficient time to have these ordered. She examines the patient and finds a normal lower extremity vascular exam, so a left osteocutaneous (skin plus bone) fibula flap is planned to replace the mandible and oral mucosa.

The following day, the cancer surgeon gets a late start because there is an educational conference that he needs to attend as the guest speaker. In the rush to schedule surgery, he also forgot to consult General Surgery to perform the endoscopic gastric tube placement, so additional time is spent finding an available surgeon to do this. Once started, he finds the neck dissection challenging due to prior radiation therapy and is concerned that the contralateral nodes may also be affected. A bilateral neck dissection is performed. The mandible resection ends up quite a bit wider than originally planned, crossing the midline.

As the cancer surgeon performs his resection, the plastic surgeon begins to harvest the fibula from the left leg. She minimizes the amount of the skin to be harvested to ease closure of the donor site. The peroneal artery (supplying the bone to be transferred) is quite small in diameter and somewhat atherosclerotic, but a Doppler confirms blood flow. The bone has callus, apparently from a prior fracture.

The cancer resection is completed around 7 pm (Fig. 19.1). *As the cancer surgeon departs, the plastic surgeon explores the neck to find suitable blood vessels to supply the flap. The left neck is quite scarred, and the branches of the external carotid artery have all been ligated close to their origin. She explores the*

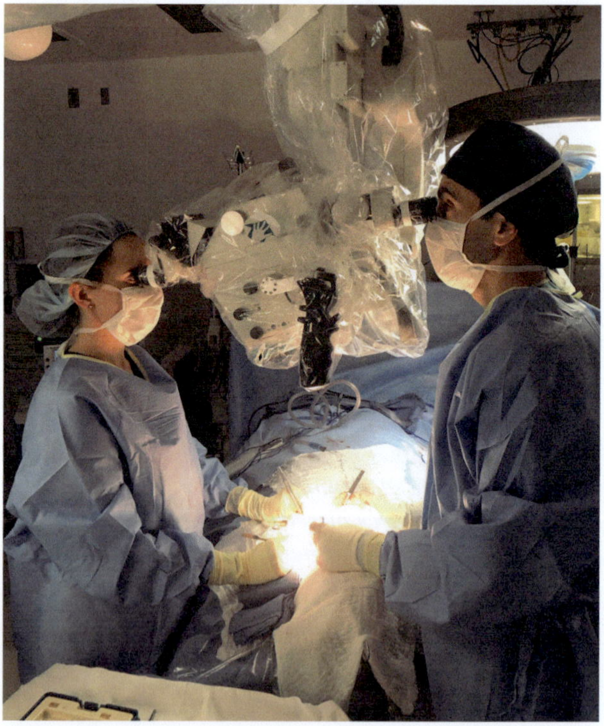

Fig. 19.1 The reconstructive dilemma following removal of the left hemi-mandible

contralateral neck and finds a suitable artery. The bone-skin flap is harvested, and the bone is cut and plated to the native remnant mandible. The vessels are found to be too short to reach the neck vessels for anastomosis. The skin paddle is also too small to replace the missing oral mucosa and external skin. As a result of these issues, a second flap must be harvested from the forearm along with some segments of vein to create "jump grafts" between the flap and its blood supply in the neck. There is a one-hour delay in getting the operating microscope into the operating room, because it was reserved for another operation that has not yet been completed. To make matters worse, the vascular anastomoses are particularly challenging due to the vascular disease in the peroneal artery. The reconstructive surgery takes most of the night, ending around 6 am. The plastic surgeon is exhausted but heads to clinic for a full day of patient visits. The patient is transferred to the Intensive Care Unit for postoperative care.

The patient's postoperative course is initially unremarkable, but he presents to clinic 8 weeks postoperatively with drainage of fluid from a hole in the skin over the mandible reconstruction. The plated jawbone is now loose and unstable, suggesting nonunion at the site of the distal fibula transferred to reconstruct the mandible. A bone scan confirms the bone adjacent to the old fracture site is dead. Another reconstruction must now be planned to replace the infected and non-viable mandible segment.

Analysis

In the rush to perform a cancer operation on a VIP patient, the surgeons in this example inadvertently donned "blinders" and abandoned their typical methodical approach to patient care that they are well trained for. The cancer surgeon went into the operation not knowing the approximate extent of the cancer excision he would have to perform, and he did not plan his day or the sequence of procedures. Communication was poor between the surgeons regarding not only the expected size of the defect, but also the need to preserve an appropriate blood supply to the transferred tissue.

While the extra time taken was an inconvenience to the cancer surgeon, the downstream effect of prolonging the reconstruction may have affected the reconstructive surgeon's judgment as well. The plastic surgeon did not examine the patient or obtain the appropriate history. Noting a prior tibia-fibula fracture would likely have prompted a more detailed workup and should have convinced the surgeon to choose the opposite fibula instead, avoiding the unhealthy bone segment. Surgical skill includes developing protocols and habitual sequences to prevent mistakes or missing details [1]. The plastic surgeon normally would have ordered a detailed 3D model of the mandible and leg to make sure the blood supply was adequate and that the bone stock could be cut to fit the anticipated defect. While each surgeon has his or her own approach, and there is considerable debate about the necessity of imaging prior to reconstructive surgery, deviating from one's own working approach lends to errors by drifting away from a tried-and-tested approach into a less methodical on-the-fly sort of decision making. Cutting corners can be a costly mistake as seen here. In hastily adding this complex case onto the operating room schedule, the need for another specialist (the general surgeon) and equipment (the operating microscope) was neglected. The prolonged ischemia time before reattaching the flap to its new blood supply (exacerbated by other delays) may also have been a contributing factor to this non-ideal outcome.

How Can We Improve Reconstructive Surgery Utilizing Human Factors Principles?

Humans are fallible, and poor time management can lead to stressful conditions made worse by exhaustion and frustration with non-ideal circumstances [2]. There are many ways to classify and analyze failure, but a common theme in the analysis of medical mistakes relates to whether errors result from inadequate planning to achieve an end goal (i.e., "mistakes") or from failure to execute a reasonable plan. There is also often consideration as to whether the unintended outcome can be attributed to an error (an unexpected result following a well-intended plan) versus a "violation," which is a deviation from an established rule of practice [3]. Our example illustrates an inadequate plan (decisions were made early despite a lack of sufficient data) and violation of normal practices (steps that should have been followed by each specialist were skipped).

Reconstructive surgery is particularly vulnerable to inadequate planning and violations. A significant percentage of reconstructive procedures are planned close to the time of their execution and with inadequate data to make fully informed choices. As the adage goes, the devil is in the details. Choosing a form of reconstruction is contingent upon many invisible factors being ideal to make the plan viable (e.g., adequate flap vessels, adequate tissue quality/volume/area, and adequate recipient vessels). Experience helps the surgeon in several ways. Understanding what problems are likely to arise, what information is needed to make decisions, and what options are most likely to succeed—these get somewhat easier with experience. One habit that contributes to experience is the adoption of mental checklists. Airline safety and operating room best practices research have proven that checklists and repetition lead to fewer *violation* type errors [4]. Teaching surgery to postgraduate trainees is also more effective when a methodical approach is demonstrated and repeated [5].

When *experience is lacking*, or whenever unusual situations arise, thorough planning becomes most critical. Part of planning is accumulating data that will come in handy when decisions must be made (such as which flap to use, which vessel to plug into, and so on). And wherever *data is lacking*, the surgeon must (1) communicate thoroughly with cooperating specialists to minimize the unexpected and (2) anticipate "worst case" scenarios and have a back-up plan for as many situations as possible.

Another important lesson to this example is understanding that the surgeon and patient exist within a hospital system that has its own moving parts. Planning and execution of a complex operation relies not just on available surgical expertise but also on the resources of time, personnel, and equipment. To be cavalier with these adjunctive components to patient care is to treat the entire endeavor as unworthy of careful planning. The butterfly effect can be applied to this notion [6]. A seemingly small misstep or miscalculation in the beginning can easily cause not just delays but *mistakes*, defined previously as adoption of an inadequate plan to achieve the end goal.

Lessons Learned/Personal Pearls

- Methodical planning is the most critical step in the execution of a complex procedure.
- Communication is vital to prevent errors of poor planning.
- Starting with a mental checklist and developing good practices through repetition are critical to establishing experience in complex problem-solving endeavors.
- Consider all the important resources needed for a successful operation, not just the surgical expertise at hand.

References

1. de Vries EN, Hollmann MW, Smorenburg SM, et al. Development and validation of the SURgical PAtient Safety System (SURPASS) checklist. BMJ Qual Saf. 2009;18:121–6.
2. Philibert I. Sleep loss and performance in residents and nonphysicians: a meta-analytic examination. Sleep. 2005;28:1392–402.
3. Reason J. Safety in the operating theatre – part 2: human error and organisational failure. Qual Saf Health Care. 2005;14:56–61.
4. Oak SN, Dave NM, Garasia MB, Parelkar SV. Surgical checklist application and its impact on patient safety in pediatric surgery. J Postgrad Med. 2015;61(2):92–4.
5. Burke CR, Mokadam NA. Repetition is the mother of skill. J Thorac Cardiovasc Surg. 2018;155(4):1694–5.
6. Oestreicher C. A history of chaos theory. Dialogues Clin Neurosci. 2007;9(3):279–89.

Human Factors in Transplant Surgery 20

Irene Kim and Tsuyoshi Todo

Overview of Transplant Surgery

Solid organ transplantation usually involves transplantation of an organ (allograft) from a human donor to a recipient, commonly necessitating immunosuppression. Historically, transplantation was reserved for patients suffering from end-stage organ failure and has evolved from kidney transplants to life-saving organs (heart, liver, lung) to improved quality-of-life organs (pancreas, hand, face, uterus, etc.).

Case Examples

When Things Can Go Wrong

A high-volume organ transplant center had accepted multiple kidney allografts for transplantation into different recipients. Two of the kidney transplant recipients were slated to receive the same blood group organ type. Routine ABO-verification was performed, as per protocol, before all performed transplants. However, at the conclusion of the operative procedures for all transplants, it was noted that two recipients had received the wrong kidney. Both patients received blood type–compatible kidney transplants but had unfortunately received the wrong kidney allografts with different HLA-tissue typing and donor profiles. It appeared that human error had led to misidentification of the organ-specific labels.

I. Kim · T. Todo (✉)
Comprehensive Transplant Center, Department of Surgery, Cedars-Sinai Medical Center, Los Angeles, CA, USA
e-mail: Irene.kim@cshs.org; Tsuyoshi.Todo@cshs.org

T. N. Cohen et al. (eds.), *Human Factors in Surgery*,
https://doi.org/10.1007/978-3-030-53127-0_20

Analysis Even though ABO-verification had taken place, surgical teams had failed to properly identify organ-specific labeling, resulting in the transplantation of the wrong allograft into the wrong recipient. This case resulted from multiple transplants occurring at the same time and an absence of a systems process to prevent this human error.

When a System Functions Well

A transplant center had three living kidney donor/recipient pairs, where the three donors were incompatible with the three recipients. In order to facilitate transplantation for all three recipients, an internal chain was planned with a three by three swap of the three donor kidneys into the different recipients. The kidney swap was planned for the same operative day, necessitating six simultaneous operating rooms, four individual surgeons, and six operating room teams. In addition, patient anonymity of all patients involved in the swap was enforced. To facilitate the coordination of multiple operating rooms and teams, a surgical "huddle" was performed prior to the start of the operative day, with donor and recipient surgical teams visually identifying one another for the handoffs. Organs were not only labeled with the United Network for Organ Sharing (UNOS)-specified organ labels but were also color coordinated to further verify organ/recipient matching (Fig. 20.1). Lastly, two dedicated procurement technicians escorted organs from one operating room to another, to add an additional layer of verification and reduce hand-off errors. Three kidney transplant recipients were successfully transplanted without error.

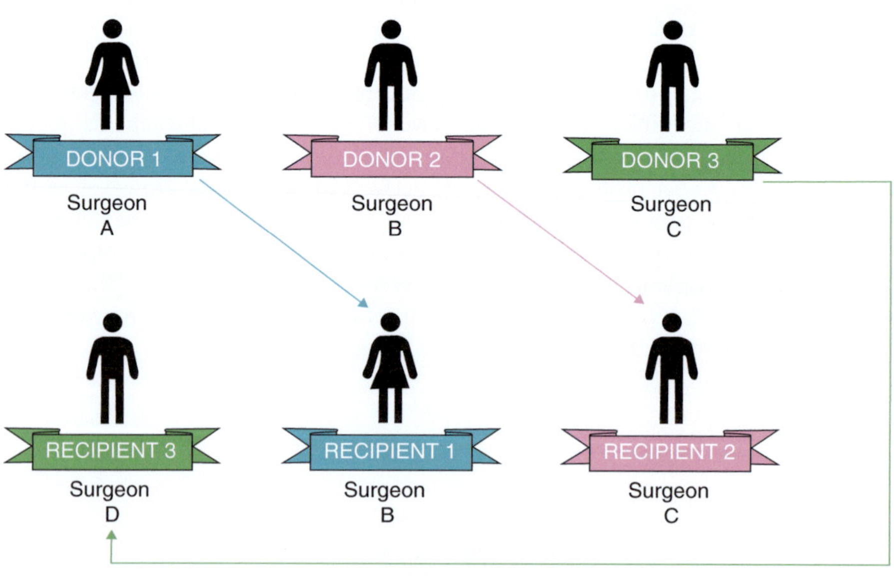

Fig. 20.1 Operative plan for actual internal kidney exchange (six patients)

Analysis Given the highly complex exchange of six separate surgical teams, multiple layers of verification were added to standard practice in order to reduce hand-off errors.

How Can We Improve Transplant Surgery Care Using Human Factor Principles?

Given the increased number of teams, surgical team members, specialized equipment, and advanced technology necessary to carry out a successful transplant surgery, it is not surprising that breakdowns in system safety and efficiency can occur. Human factors interventions will reduce disruptions that lead to errors in transplant surgery. Regulatory requirements for transplant centers established critical elements for organ transplant center certification. Despite these certifications, there are many opportunities for systems breakdowns, leading to organ loss and even patient death. Standardization of practices as a result of systematic reviews from the Institute of Medicine (IOM), University HealthSystem Consortium (UHC), and other organizations led to best practices and, in some cases, new requirements for transplant programs. For example, in 2011, Organ Procurement and Transplantation Network/United Network for Organ Sharing (OPTN/UNOS) ratified a bylaw in 2011, requiring all liver transplant centers to appoint a Director of Liver Transplant Anesthesia based on set criteria to mitigate variation of the anesthesia component in liver transplantation [1].

Communication

Surgical team members communicate in several ways, including face-to-face conversations, text messages, e-mails, notes documented in the electronic health record (EHR), and through the use of labeling. Unfortunately, data labeling is not always an accurate way of communicating (as documented during the first case study). Data published by the Organ Procurement and Transplantation Network (OPTN) and the United Network for Organ Sharing (UNOS) nearly 10 years ago found that labeling errors accounted for nearly 40% of all reported errors in transplant centers [2]. Friedman and Lee (2006) developed six steps for confirming the organ and ABO identification to ensure patient safety and prevent liability for the transplant team and the facility involved when a mislabeled organ is identified. The six steps include the following: (1) query host organ procurement organization (OPO) to identify error source; (2) request OPO documentation of nature of error; (3) verify ABO type of blood sample accompanying organ; (4) obtain administrative approval; (5) obtain legal approval; and (6) disclose nature of error and clarification steps to patient/family [3]. While these six steps are useful in determining how to address mislabeled organs, it is important to identify solutions and interventions aimed to reduce the mislabeling event in the first place.

Communication failures can also occur during face-to-face interactions when handing off a patient between two care teams. Steinberger and colleagues (2009) explored the use of the Failure Mode and Effects Analysis (FMEA) method to conduct a risk analysis surrounding communication breakdowns, involving the handoff of transplant patients [4]. FMEA is a proactive and predictive approach that looks at a process and attempts to identify all the ways in which that process could go wrong, the likelihood that the failure or defect would be detected, and the significance of the impact on performance or safety [5]. The team identified three major human factors and workload considerations to improve upon: cognitive load, fatigue, and time demands/production pressure. A list of actionable items was then developed to improve system safety and mitigate errors in this process. For example, with respect to cognitive load, a structured "organ map" or standardized checklist was developed so that transplant coordinators could track the status of specific donor–recipient matches.

Teamwork

Transplantation should be performed in designated operating rooms that allow teams of surgeons, anesthesiologists, perfusionists, nurses, and technicians the opportunity to work together in an environment conducive to communication and coordination. Often times, team members need tools in order to coordinate more effectively. In transplant surgery, tools such as a surgical checklist and universal time-outs can be useful for improving safety and efficiency. Consider, for example, a "Surgical Checklist" that standardizes the extensive pretransplant, perioperative, and postoperative clinical care required for transplant surgery (Table 20.1).

Additionally, the "universal time-out" is a well-known, pre-surgical practice used to minimize errors by ensuring that the entire team is in agreement about the patient; the scheduled procedure; the surgical site; and other patient, operative, or environmental concerns [6]. Time-outs can be particularly useful in transplant surgery and include additional discussion points surrounding confirmation of donor and recipient blood types and a discussion on any antirejection medications. Because of the value of confirming these points, we have developed a unique time-out board to help ensure that our teams consistently have a shared understanding of the patient, cross-clamp time, blood type verification, and special equipment (Fig. 20.2).

Individuals with disciplines outside of the traditional team can also be leveraged to enhance communication, teamwork, and safety. Musgrave and colleagues (2013) conducted a study to explore the impact of pharmacists on the medication reconciliation process in transplant surgery. The authors noted that transplant recipients are at a higher risk for medication errors than many other patient populations, as a transplant recipient can receive nine or more new medications in addition to their medications taken prior to their transplant surgery. During the prospective period, researchers observed a total of 191 errors made on discharge medication reconciliation; however, pharmacists prevented 119 of these errors. Comparison to a

Table 20.1 Surgical checklist

Pre-transplant
Organ donation process flow (from www.organdonor.gov) 1. Donor registration 2. Medical care of potential donor 3. Brain death testing 4. OPO 5. Authorizing donation 6. Organ matching 7. Organ recovery and transportation 8. Organ transplantation
Patient process (from www.pkdcure.org) 1. Organ failure -> evaluation for organ transplant 2. Waitlist acceptance -> registration on national list 3. Building support system 4. Waiting period 5. Transplant 6. Post-operative care
Intraoperative considerations 1. Operating room team (a) Surgical Team (b) Anesthesia Team (c) Nursing (d) Surgical Technician (e) Perfusion Team (f) Dialysis Nurse 2. Size of Operating room (a) Surgical instruments (b) Anesthesia machine (c) Perfusion devices (d) Blood product storage (e) Back Table 3. Blood product verification 4. ABO – Organ Verification 5. Pre-operative Time Out
Post-operative care 1. Inpatient care: Protocols for immunosuppression 2. Outpatient care: Protocols for follow up and team management 3. Long-term follow up

retrospective data sample (when pharmacists were not part of the care team) identified 430 errors, none of which were prevented at the time of discharge when pharmacists were involved with medication reconciliation [7].

Equipment and Technology

Operating rooms must accommodate the equipment challenges unique to transplantation, for example, liver transplantation may require intraoperative continuous renal replacement therapy (CRRT). This continuous dialysis machine takes up a

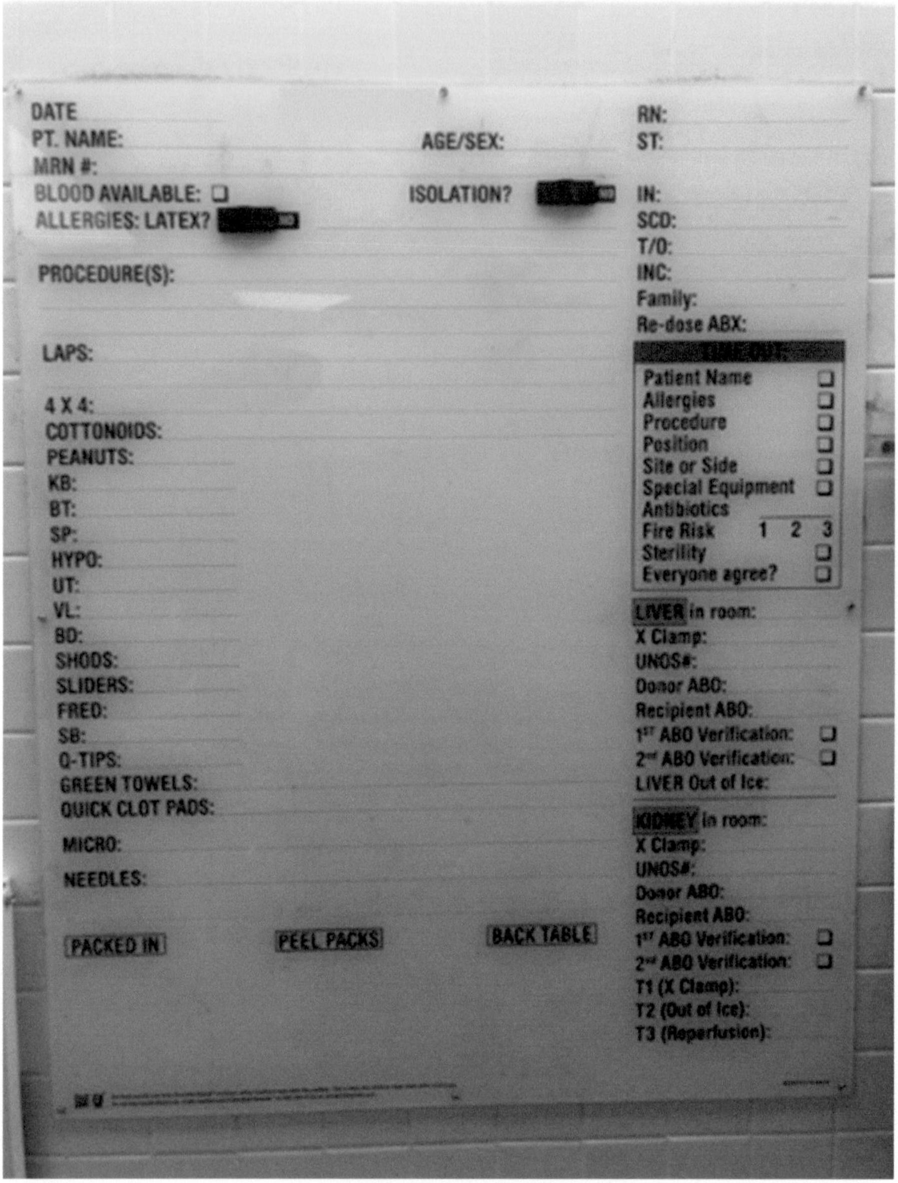

Fig. 20.2 Use of preoperative organ-specific "time-out" board

considerable amount of space and requires the support of a dialysis nurse to operate the machine in the room during the entire case.

Efficiency and Safety

Human factors interventions can help alleviate challenges in areas outside of the operating room that can have an impact on surgical patients. For example, consider challenges surrounding bed availability for incoming patients scheduled to receive an organ. Inefficient patient flow can cause unique challenges for transplantation. Once explanted, an organ has a limited time that it will be viable before transplantation. If an organ becomes available when there are no hospital beds to immediately admit its recipient, challenges arise as the recipient cannot be admitted for preoperative preparation. Given that well-trained teams can work together independent of the location of the available hospital beds, stable kidney transplant patients can be managed in the post-anesthesia care unit (PACU) by the same team that manages the patient in a floor bed. This focus on team rather than bed location reduces the pressure to open a bed in a full hospital and improve efficiency and safety for the transplant patient.

We developed a multidisciplinary team to create a test of change to improve inpatient bed availability and reduce delays for kidney transplant. The test of change involved three interventions: (1) having kidney transplant patients bypass the inpatient unit and go directly to the preoperative area before surgery, (2) introducing an order-set that defaulted to STAT labs, STAT-portable chest X-ray, and STAT dialysis (if applicable), and (3) signing the patient consent in pre-op instead of the inpatient unit. This initiative required close collaboration with multiple process stakeholders, including nursing, pre-op/PACU staff, OR leadership, transplant coordinators, surgeons, anesthesiologists, admissions, and patient placement teams. Overall, this intervention also helped improve efficiency by minimizing patient transport and handoffs from the floor, pre-op area, and radiology and cut down on the wait time for transporters.

Lessons Learned/Personal Pearls

- Standardization of practices in high-volume transplant centers is a common theme, and anecdotally, members of transplant centers report, "All members practice and perform transplantation in the same way, every time."
- Written protocols allow for resource documentation for all transplant team members to refer to, especially when practice discrepancies arise. There

are protocols written for virtually all aspects listed in Table 20.1. As in compliance with UNOS policy, we have a dedicated quality team that manages these protocols.

- Enhanced communication tools such as the universal time-out board may help team members maintain a shared mental model regarding the patient, equipment, technology, and the operation, thereby ensuring patient safety.
- Transplant surgery can benefit from the inclusion of multidisciplinary team members at all care points.

References

1. Organ procurement and transplantation network bylaws (2020). https://optn.transplant.hrsa.gov/media/1201/optn_bylaws.pdf.
2. Report to the Board of Directors. Richmond, VA: 2010. OPTN/UNOS Operations and Safety Committee.
3. Friedman AL, Lee KC, Lee GD. Errors in ABO labeling of deceased donor kidneys: case reports and approach to ensuring patient safety. Am J Transplant. 2007;7(2):480–3.
4. Steinberger DM, Douglas SV, Kirschbaum MS. Use of failure mode and effects analysis for proactive identification of communication and handoff failures from organ procurement to transplantation. Prog Transplant. 2009;19(3):208–14.
5. Alban RF, Anania EC, Cohen TN, et al. Performance improvement in surgery. Curr Probl Surg. 2019;56(6):204–8.
6. Paramesh AS. What's new in the transplant OR? AORN J. 2013;97(4):435–47.
7. Musgrave CR, Pilch NA, Taber DJ, et al. Improving transplant patient safety through pharmacist discharge medication reconciliation. Am J Transplant. 2013;13(3):796–801.

21 Exploring Human Factors in Trauma

Eric J. Ley and Tara N. Cohen

What Is Trauma

Trauma involves life-threatening, critical injuries where there is a question of immediate survival. During trauma care, a team of highly specialized individuals including surgeons, nurses, and technicians must work as efficiently as possible to increase the likelihood of a patient's survival.

Case Study

To better understand how human factors can lead to a well-designed system that provides the highest possible care, or alternatively prevents catastrophe, here are two case stories.

When Things Can Go Wrong

A high-level trauma was called due to the report of a hypotensive patient with a stab wound to the left chest. The time between the trauma page and patient arrival was minimal and no equipment was ready when the patient arrived. The trauma surgeon and the emergency department (ED) attending had not worked together before this evening. When the patient arrived, the emergency medical services (EMS) were delivering chest compression due to the loss of pulses during transport. The ED attending stated that per protocol this patient did not meet criteria to receive additional care and resuscitation should cease. At that time, the nursing staff stopped connecting the monitor, and the clinicians briefly stopped chest compressions,

E. J. Ley (✉) · T. N. Cohen
Cedars-Sinai Medical Center, Los Angeles, CA, USA
e-mail: Eric.Ley@cshs.org; Tara.cohen@cshs.org

T. N. Cohen et al. (eds.), *Human Factors in Surgery*,
https://doi.org/10.1007/978-3-030-53127-0_21

resulting in a disruption such that the patient was no longer receiving any care. Conversely, the trauma attending then expressed that per protocol, care should continue for the patient and requested a thoracotomy tray. A brief discussion then occurred between team members regarding the appropriate action and who was in charge. Care then resumed; the patient was connected to a monitor where pulseless electrical activity (PEA) was noted, which indicated that the patient's heart was attempting to beat, but it could not due to compression from blood around the heart. The patient was intubated, and a thoracotomy revealed pericardial tamponade. The pericardial sac was opened to evacuate the blood. With open heart massage, the heart began to beat but a sustained rhythm could not be obtained. The patient was taken to the operating room (OR) where attempts to resuscitate were unsuccessful.

Analysis: Preparation prior to arrival in order to huddle with the team and ready equipment did not occur, which led to a lack of necessary equipment and assignment of roles. This case lacked leadership, and as a result, team performance suffered. To compound the challenges to the team, the trauma and ED attendings had not previously worked together. A protocol for care after penetrating trauma to the chest may have assisted with the care.

When a System Functions Well

During a grocery store strike in Los Angeles, the tensions were high between those who continued to work and others who chose to strike. On an early weekday morning while an employee walked to work, an associate stabbed him in the chest. He was able to call for help, and EMS quickly transported him to the hospital. The trauma team was notified and ready at bedside with a chest tube and thoracotomy tray. Upon arrival, the patient presented with a 2-cm stab wound in his left chest. His blood pressure was 95/50 and heart rate was 110. The chest X-ray (CXR) determined that the left lung was up and the focused assessment with sonography in trauma (FAST) ultrasound indicated that there was blood around the heart. The attending trauma surgeon rapidly communicated with the OR to prepare the surgical team. As the patient was readied for transport, the monitor was faulty, so the decision was made to transport the patient without a monitor. As the patient was wheeled out of the trauma bay, the resident stated that he could not feel a pulse, and so the patient returned to the trauma bay and was placed back on the ED monitor. The patient was in PEA due to tamponade, so a thoracotomy was performed with the equipment that was already present, and the blood around the heart was rapidly evacuated. The laceration in the heart was closed in the ED, and the patient was then taken to the OR for definitive closure and discharged in 4 days.

Analysis: Given the team had a history of working together, there was open communication among members about the changing exam and the coordination with the OR staff. Role assignment was important such that the trauma attending valued the resident's observation regarding the changing exam. The malfunctioning equipment could have led to catastrophe, but the ability to overcome the broken monitor is a characteristic of a high-reliability system.

How Can We Improve Trauma Care Using Human Factor Principles?

Surgeons are proficient in managing trauma systems in order to deliver rapid treatment and save lives (Fig. 21.1) [1]. Unfortunately, even the most talented surgeon can encounter a scenario where a systemic breakdown causes catastrophe. For example, the request for massive transfusion is highly important and sometimes dependent on a junior member of the team. If the intern who hears the request for massive transfusion is then sidetracked by another request for an arterial blood gas (ABG), the rapid delivery of blood products may be delayed. How can the surgeon become an expert in managing this system? In high-risk environments, the system must improve around its users rather than forcing the users to fit the system. Improvements in the delivery of trauma require an understanding of the many, varied components of the trauma system. What are policies in place that guide the care? Communication and coordination are key. Teamwork with role assignment is essential. This chapter will expand upon how one trauma system was improved through human factors insights.

James Reason's Swiss Cheese model of Accident Investigation can be used to conceptualize why medical errors may occur and provides insights for error avoidance (Fig. 21.2) [2]. For example, consider a patient in the intensive care unit (ICU) with an internal jugular cordis catheter. Let's say that a new intern erroneously removes the catheter in a patient who is sitting in a chair, resulting in a venous air embolism that leads to the patient's death. The solution in this unsafe system often involves placing the blame on the individual who committed the error. Unfortunately, this approach fails to identify and mitigate potential threats to patient safety and is unlikely to protect the system from this type of error again. However, if the new intern erroneously removes the catheter in a safe system, there would be many layers of protection in place to mitigate this and other types of serious adverse events. For example, up-to-date protocols that are widely disseminated can help prevent drift in care that leads to complications. Training and supervision

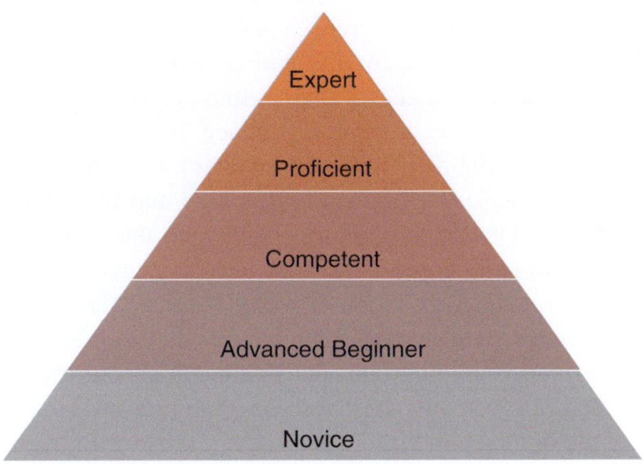

Fig. 21.1 Five-stage model of mental activities involved in direct skill acquisition. (Adapted from Dreyfus and Dreyfus [1])

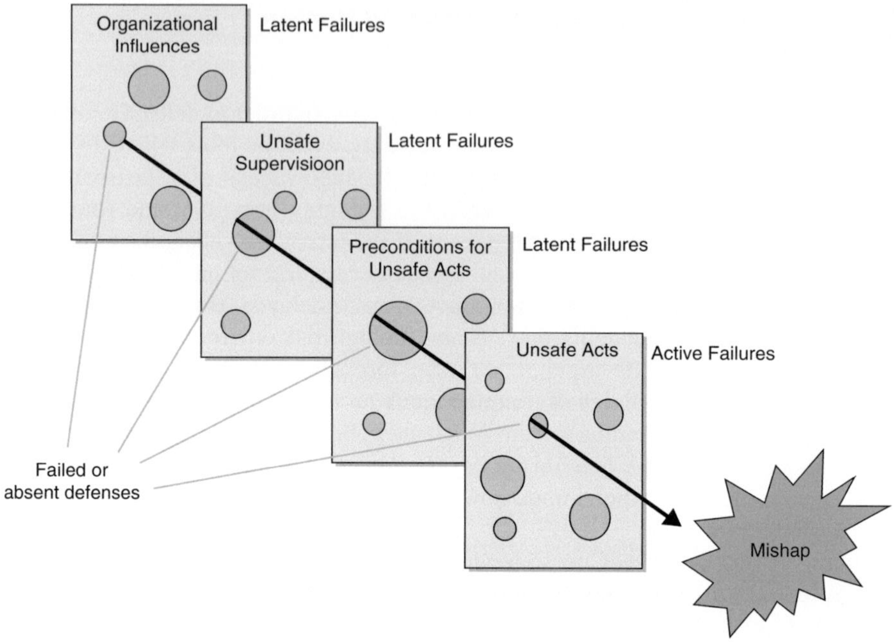

Fig. 21.2 James Reason's Swiss Cheese model of accident causation. (Adapted from Reason [2])

of inexperienced physicians leads to better habits. High-quality communication consisting of check-backs and closed-loop communication would be encouraged; perhaps, the intern could have discussed the plan for cordis removal with the nursing staff, who would have guided the patient back to bed. When there are breakdowns in these layers that protect against threats to the system, failures can cascade into serious harm.

One challenge when adapting to a more modern perspective on systems-focused care is that the importance placed upon a single leader is reduced. Comparing a traditional perspective of trauma care delivery to a modern systems perspective demonstrates many differences in thinking. With a traditional perspective, the focus is on errors and procedural violations among the individuals. Unsafe acts arise from aberrant mental processes such as inattentiveness, lack of good judgment, forgetfulness, recklessness, or even negligence. Interventions are directly aimed at reducing unwanted variability in human behavior. Common methods include retraining, disciplinary measures, or even termination and litigation. When taken to the extreme, errors are viewed as a moral issue, with the belief that bad things such as errors happen to bad people. With a modern systems perspective of trauma care, humans are fallible, and errors are expected, even in the best organizations. Disruptions in care are consequences of deficient processes and/or system failures. Consistency in performance is important, but flexibility is also invaluable during dynamic operations. Improvements are based on changing working conditions rather than changing the human condition. Importantly, those with the highest level of technical skill and the best intentions can and do make errors. Thus, attempts to reduce errors should focus on how and why the system failed.

One human factors intervention that may be utilized to improve a high-risk system is a checklist. The checklist may reduce errors by mandating specific steps within a high-risk environment. The aviation industry has successfully employed safety checklists during high-workload times that are likely to encounter disruptions in the flow of safe operations. The surgical community also has examined the use of a checklist to improve patient safety through team safety and consistency of care. The challenge with an intervention such as a checklist is that an understanding of the system is required prior to introducing the checklist. Some health-care systems may benefit from a checklist, while others may not. The surgical safety checklist (Fig. 21.3) is one example of a checklist that may work in one system but not another [3]. Haynes et al. published in the New England Journal of Medicine (NEJM) the impact of the introduction of a surgical safety checklist and demonstrated that at the eight study hospitals, there was a reduction in mortality (1.5% vs. 0.8%, $p < 0.01$) and complications (11.0% vs. 7.0%, $p < 0.01$). In contrast, the introduction of surgical safety checklist at 101 Canadian hospitals demonstrated no difference in mortality or complications (Fig. 21.4) [4]. Understanding why one intervention such as a checklist impacts one hospital system but not another requires additional data. In the Haynes paper, the eight hospitals were analyzed individually, and variable improvement was noted. Hospital Site 1, for example, completed 94.1% of the six safety indicators before the introduction of the checklist and 94.2% after its introduction. The checklist was unlikely to improve this site, and it is possible that its introduction led to disruptions in care. The 101 Canadian hospitals may have similarly observed little

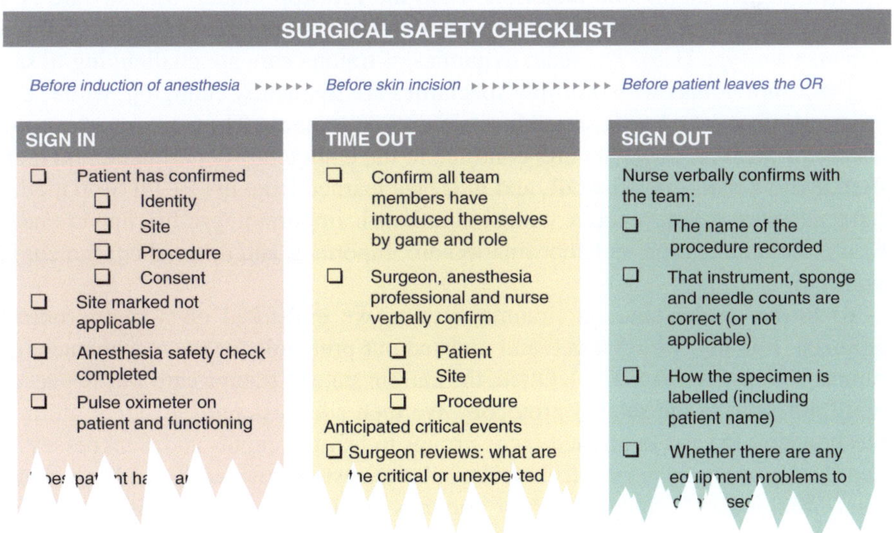

Fig. 21.3 The surgical safety checklist. (Adapted from Haynes et al. [3])

Site No. *	No. of Patients Enrolled		% Objective Airway Evaluation Performed (N=7688)		% Pulse Oximeter Used (N=7688)		% Two Peripheral or One Central IV Catheter Present at Incision When EBL ≥ 500 ml (N=953)		% Prophylactic Antibiotics Given Appropriately (N=6802)		% Oral Confirmation of Patient's Identity and Operative Site (N=7688)		% Sponge Count Completed (N=7572)		% All six Safety Indicators Performed (N=7688)	
	Before	After	Before	After	Before	After	Before	After	Before	After	Before	After	Before	After	Before	After
1	524	598	97.0	98.5	100.0	100.0	95.7	83.6	98.1	96.9	100.0	100.0	98.9	100.0	94.1	94.2
2	357	351	72.0	75.8	97.5	98.6	78.8	61.3	56.9	76.9	9.5	97.2	100.0	100.0	3.6	55.3
5	370	330	6.2	0.0	68.9	91.2	7.6	2.7	29.8	96.2	0.0	86.1	0.0	92.4	0.0	0.0
8	444	584	0.5	94.0	99.3	99.5	68.8	57.1	18.2	77.6	16.4	98.8	61.3	70.0	0.0	51.7
Total	3733	3955	64.0	77.2	93.6	96.8	58.1	63.2	56.1	82.6	54.4	92.3	84.6	94.6	34.2	56.7
P value			<0.001		<0.001		0.32		<0.001		<0.001		<0.001		<0.001	

** Only 4 of the 8 sites were included in this table. Totals and P values are based on full data set*

Fig. 21.4 Selected process measures before and after checklist implementation, according to site. (Adapted from Haynes et al. [3])

benefit related to the introduction of a surgical safety checklist because of little improvement in the process measures.

With trauma care, the introduction of interventions requires a thoughtful approach with a comprehensive understanding of the trauma system. Rather than depending on a simple solution, such as a checklist, to benefit every trauma center, our trauma center embarked on a detailed analysis of the trauma flow, followed by targeted interventions based upon what we learned during the initial learning phase.

We approached our analysis by comparing our trauma center to another high-risk environment, Formula 1 (F1) racing. Specifically, we focused on the Pit Stop portion of the race. During a typical Pit Stop, the multidisciplinary team must come together to change four tires and refuel the car as quickly as possible. When high-performance race cars head to the Pit Stop, the turnaround time is often under 5 seconds. The race would be changed significantly if a given pit stop was not so well orchestrated. If crew were in the incorrect positions or failing to communicate effectively, life-threatening catastrophe could easily occur due to working with highly flammable materials. Like the Pit Stop model, trauma care is a complex interaction between team members to provide emergent care to unstable patients (see Fig. 21.5). The team dynamics of trauma care are challenging to say the least. Individuals with multiple specialties are frequently changing, while several handoffs must take place within various environments. The pit stops of trauma care begin with prehospital care, continue to the emergency department, and then often involve radiology, the OR, and ICU. We learned from the F1 Pit Stop model that leadership is key, practice with simulations is important, pre-briefing are necessary, communication and coordination are important, and optimal equipment is required.

To further understand our trauma system, we embarked on a multipronged approach. Initially, we reviewed and updated our protocols for the management of trauma patients (see Fig. 21.6). Often, the current state of trauma care was not accurately reflected in the related protocols. We then administered the safety attitude questionnaire [5] and facilitated focus groups to learn strengths and weaknesses as identified by doctors, nurses, technicians, pharmacists, social works, and case managers. Weaknesses included a lack of briefings in clinical areas and failure to know the names of individuals working together. Strengths included reliable equipment

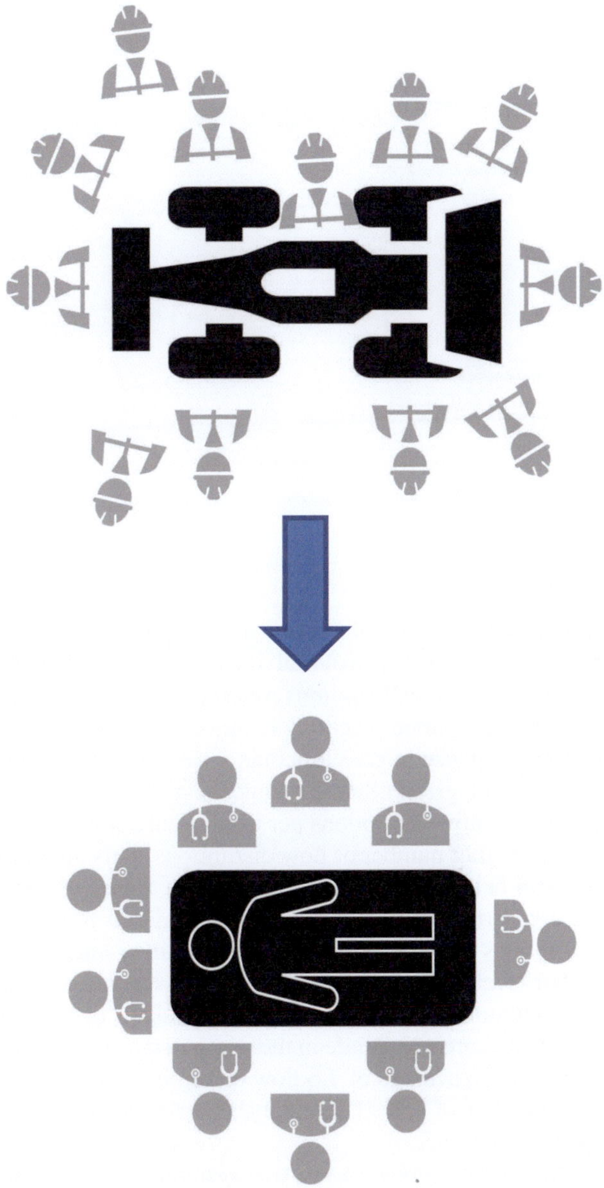

Fig. 21.5 Application of the Pit Stop model to trauma care

and a common perception that individuals would feel safe if they were being treated at the trauma center as a patient.

We then utilized trained observers to follow patients from the ED trauma bay, through radiology and if indicated to the OR, ICU, and/or ward. The observers recorded the number and category of flow disruptions (i.e., any instance where there was a deviation in the natural progression of the task) [6]. Identified flow disruptions

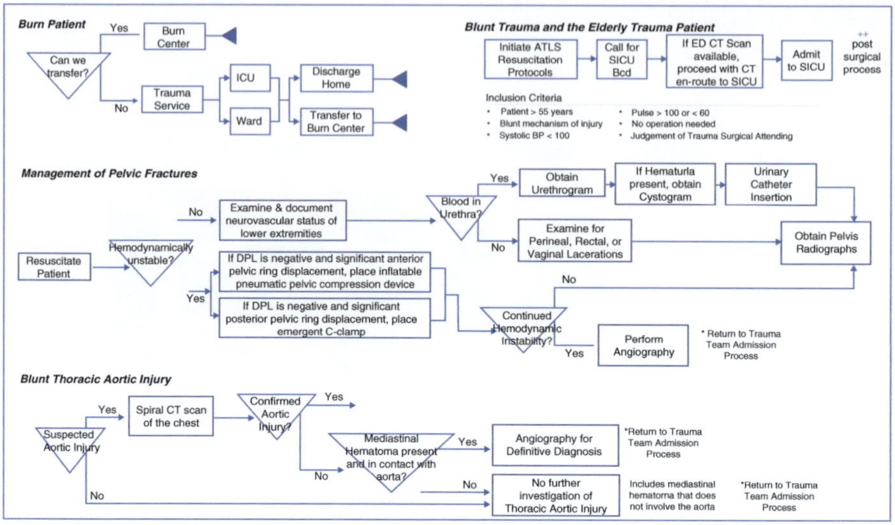

Fig. 21.6 Protocols for the management of trauma patients

were categorized into the following categories: communication, coordination, environment, equipment, external interruptions, patient factors, technical skills, and training. The flow disruptions were also assigned an impact score from 0 to 3 (0: no impact (e.g., phone ringing); 1: minimal impact, no pause (e.g., repeat communication); 2: pause in care less than 2 minutes (e.g., equipment malfunction); and 3: pause in care greater than 2 minutes (e.g., consultant not available)) [7]. Overall, the number of flow disruptions per trauma case was 20.4, and the more severe traumas led to a higher number of flow disruptions. This finding refuted the belief that teams perform better with higher acuity cases. Here, we saw that more flow disruptions were reported when a more severely injured trauma patient was observed. Flow disruptions were more likely to occur during care of trauma patients who required higher level of care in the OR or the surgical intensive care unit (SICU).

Additionally, we conducted a sub-analysis of the workflow during radiology for trauma patients [8]. While in the computed tomography (CT) scanner, we found that there was an average of 7.6 flow disruptions per patient, which were largely due to coordination of care. Ultimately, this contributed to an average time of 30.5 min spent in imaging.

After being sure we had a true systemic understanding of our trauma system, we then embarked on developing targeted interventions. This is in direct contrast to introducing an intervention such as a checklist, as discussed with the surgical safety checklist earlier, and expecting improvement with little understanding of the system.

The interventions chosen were considered with input from experts in trauma care, human factors, and quality improvement. Each was based upon what was learned from reviewing the process maps, results from the safety attitude questionnaire, and focus groups' feedback, as well as the observed flow disruptions.

Many of the targeted interventions were studied in simulation or small trials prior to full implementation. Using maps of provider movement during high-level traumas, we standardized the trauma bays so that the equipment in each bay was in similar areas. The role of huddles prior to the patient arrival were studied in a limited trial, which demonstrated that the time to the first CXR or lab blood draw were reduced when the huddle occurred prior to the patient arrival. We also evaluated the implementation of a headset to improve communication in mock trauma scenarios; however, little improvement in efficiency or quality of communication was noted, so the headsets were not included in the final interventions. In addition, all residents received teamwork training that was delivered over 3 weeks. A simple CT checklist consisting of A (airway secure), B (bring blood), and C (consults called) was introduced. A medication pack including medication for sedation, loss of airway, and code blue events for transporting patients was made available. Transport monitors were updated, and broken monitors were removed. Finally, a standardized whiteboard presented prehospital information to assist with planning prior to patient arrival.

After the targeted interventions were evaluated and implemented, we embarked on a second observer period where we captured the number and category of flow disruptions to better understand how our system changed due to the interventions. We learned that patients going to the OR had a net reduction of 11.9 flow disruptions and those going to CT had a net reduction of 2.0 flow disruptions. The mean time in the ED for high-level trauma decreased from 60 minutes to 30 minutes, and for low level-trauma, the decrease was from 65 minutes to 45 minutes. Additionally, our interventions led to a reduced length of stay for high-level traumas [7].

Lessons Learned/Personal Pearls

- Improving any process requires an in-depth understanding of the system prior to interventions.
- Design the system around the users rather than forcing users to fit the system.
- Traditional approaches often fall short when used to improve performance; given the opportunity, one should always choose a more systemic approach.
- It is important to trial all interventions, especially those involving the introduction of complex technology.
- Input from frontline providers at the "sharp" end of the system can provide helpful insights into the current state of the system.

References

1. Dreyfus SE, Dreyfus HL. A five-stage model of the mental activities involved in directed skill acquisition. Berkeley: California Univ Berkeley Operations Research Center; 1980.
2. Reason J. Human error. Cambridge: Cambridge University Press; 1990.

3. Haynes AB, Weiser TG, Berry WR, Lipsitz SR, Breizat A-HS, Dellinger EP, et al. A surgical safety checklist to reduce morbidity and mortality in a global population. N Engl J Med. 2009;360(5):491–9.
4. Urbach DR, Govindarajan A, Saskin R, Wilton AS, Baxter NN. Introduction of surgical safety checklists in Ontario, Canada. N Engl J Med. 2014;370(11):1029–38.
5. Sexton JB, Helmreich RL, Neilands TB, Rowan K, Vella K, Boyden J, et al. The Safety Attitudes Questionnaire: psychometric properties, benchmarking data, and emerging research. BMC Health Serv Res. 2006;6(1):44.
6. Wiegmann DA, ElBardissi AW, Dearani JA, Daly RC, Sundt Iii TM. Disruptions in surgical flow and their relationship to surgical errors: an exploratory investigation. Surgery. 2007;142(5):658–65.
7. Shouhed D, Blocker R, Gangi A, Ley E, Blaha J, Margulies D, et al. Flow disruptions during trauma care. World J Surg. 2014;38(2):314–21.
8. Blocker RC, Shouhed D, Gangi A, Ley E, Blaha J, Gewertz BL, et al. Barriers to trauma patient care associated with CT scanning. J Am Coll Surg. 2013;217(1):135–41.

Identifying Opportunities to Enhance Thoracic Surgery Using Human Factors

22

Deven C. Patel and Douglas Z. Liou

What Is Thoracic Surgery?

Thoracic surgery refers to the care of patients with surgical diseases of the chest, including the heart, great vessels, lungs, airway, esophagus, mediastinum, chest wall, and diaphragm. Acuity in the specialty can range from a type A aortic dissection requiring emergent cardiac surgery to a planned elective resection for lung cancer. Given the inherent challenges of thoracic anatomy as well as the complexity of performing surgery in the chest, operations routinely require a multidisciplinary team. Thus, effective coordination, communication, and problem-solving are essential to ensure patient safety and optimal surgical outcomes.

Case Study

The following case illustrates how human factors issues such as case delays, and mental states such as frustration, can disrupt a routine thoracic surgical oncology operation and potentially result in unnecessary major surgery.

D. C. Patel
Division of General Surgery, Department of Surgery,
Cedars-Sinai Medical Center, Los Angeles, CA, USA

Division of Thoracic Surgery, Department of Cardiothoracic Surgery,
Stanford University, Stanford, CA, USA
e-mail: dcpatel@stanford.edu

D. Z. Liou (✉)
Division of Thoracic Surgery, Department of Cardiothoracic Surgery,
Stanford University, Stanford, CA, USA
e-mail: dliou@stanford.edu

T. N. Cohen et al. (eds.), *Human Factors in Surgery*,
https://doi.org/10.1007/978-3-030-53127-0_22

When Delays Lead to Distractions

A patient with a 3.5-cm central biopsy–proven adenocarcinoma of the right upper lobe is scheduled for mediastinoscopy for staging, followed by a robot-assisted right upper lobectomy—presuming the mediastinal lymph nodes are negative for metastasis on frozen section. The case was delayed for 2 hours due to new personnel in the operating room (OR) who were unfamiliar with the robot setup for thoracic procedures. The attending surgeon was distressed when the case began and rushed through the preoperative briefing. Importantly, he did not specify to his new team that proceeding with the lobectomy is predicated on negative lymph nodes from the mediastinoscopy. The mediastinoscopy begins in routine fashion; however, the surgeon is curt with the scrub tech and circulating nurse as he passes off and names each lymph node sample. Periodically grumbling that they are "so behind" due to the "unacceptable" late start as he works quickly to "make up time." The scrub tech and nurse fall behind with labeling the specimens without communicating to the surgeon. The surgeon continues to place sample after sample in front of the scrub tech, shouting out names of each, as he moves to the next biopsy. Struggling to keep up, the scrub tech misses the name of several samples, so he sets them aside and plans to clarify with the surgeon after all samples are taken.

As the surgeon begins to close the neck incision, the scrub tech asks for clarification on the samples that have not been sent to pathology yet. At this moment, however, the surgeon notices the robot is positioned incorrectly for lobectomy and demands that this is fixed immediately by someone who "knows what they are doing." As soon as the incision is closed, the circulating nurse and scrub tech scramble to find help. During repositioning of the robot and patient for lobectomy, the surgeon calls the charge nurse into the room and requests a new surgical team. After all is settled and the pathologist confirms the provided samples that were sent demonstrate no lymph node metastasis, the surgeon begins the lobectomy with his new team. It is not until the surgeon is well into the hilar dissection and has already divided the pulmonary vein when the new scrub tech notices that the unsent lymph node samples are waiting on the sterile field to be properly labeled and sent off to pathology for frozen.

Analysis

Thoracic surgery is heavily dependent on an effective multidisciplinary team to communicate and coordinate care for each patient. In this scenario, the thoracic surgeon performs a mediastinoscopy and sends lymph node samples to the pathologist for frozen section analysis. Clinically, this action is incredibly important, as the discovery of cancer within the mediastinal nodes dictate whether the patient should have primary surgery versus induction therapy followed by surgery. In this scenario, several lymph node samples were left out of the pathologic evaluation due to a variety of distracting factors, resulting in incomplete staging prior to starting the lung resection.

The process of invasive mediastinal staging in thoracic oncology is highly dependent on human factors, as the process involves several handoffs with the potential for communication failures. During mediastinoscopy, the surgeon collects and gives samples of nodal tissue to the scrub tech, who is then responsible for ensuring all samples are accounted for and labeled appropriately by the circulating nurse. All samples must then be passed off to a member of the pathology department, who is responsible for collecting and transporting the samples, while relaying the clinical question put forth by the surgeon for the pathologist. Next, the pathologist is responsible for closely examining the tissue and providing an accurate response to the surgeon. Similar to the childhood game of telephone, the potential for breakdowns in communication are many. An error anywhere in this communication chain can potentially lead to inaccurate staging and treatment. From a human factors perspective, the abovementioned case demonstrates several system vulnerabilities that make errors in this scenario possible.

Team familiarity is incredibly important for a high-functioning group of individuals to work and communicate effectively. Communication is greatly hampered when emotional factors arise due to unforeseen issues, such as case delays and new unfamiliar personnel. Practicing and proper implementation of a standardized protocol during safety moments can help mitigate the impact of unexpected emotional distractions. The rushed attitude of the surgeon prohibited a formal introduction of all team members in the OR during the case. Additionally, an approach commonly adopted by surgeons is to review the surgical plan during the preoperative briefing. For instance, the surgeon in the abovementioned case was aware of the several new members in the OR and should have emphasized the importance of obtaining accurate nodal staging, as this alone would dictate whether they proceed with the major portion of the operation. These few minutes taken to communicate the surgeon's plan of action to all team members also serves as an opportunity for questions regarding patient coordination, equipment, and logistics to be answered. Additionally, as the surgeon is handing off samples to the scrub tech, the use of closed-loop communication would serve as a safety measure to ensure accurate labeling of the samples. Communication between pathologist and surgeon in this scenario is also important to note. Rather than sending the message that "all samples" were negative for cancer, reporting the names of the specimens that were received along with the pathology result of each sample can serve as another layer of safety to check that all intended samples were analyzed and accounted for.

Familiarity with the procedure being conducted also serves a role in helping the system run seamlessly and safely. In the case above involving cervical mediastinoscopy, the surgeon's normal thoracic surgery scrub tech and circulating nurse might have noticed that not all the standard five mediastinal nodal stations for this procedure (i.e., stations 2R, 4R, 2L, 4L, and 7) were sent to pathology. Familiarity with this procedure may have led one of the team members to alert the surgeon that certain specimens which are typically sent have not been accounted for in this particular case, thus allowing the error to be rectified before any clinical consequences occur.

Organizational measures can also be taken to prevent human error. For example, the use of a sterile sample board (Fig. 22.1) with preexisting labels can be placed

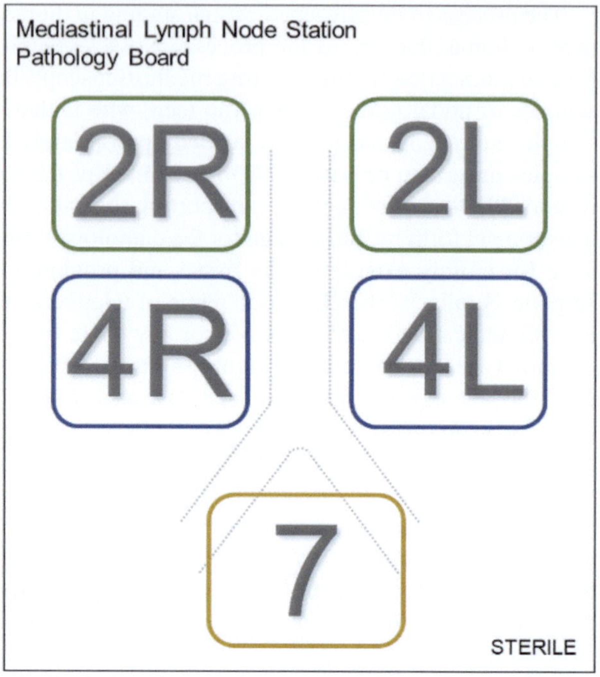

Fig. 22.1 Example of a sterile sample board for the surgeon to directly place lymph node tissue samples based on corresponding nodal station. The board would then be sent directly to the pathology department

next to the surgeon so that the tissue samples are directly placed according to the correct label. The board can then be handed off to the circulating nurse. Moreover, an organizational issue of the system was the personnel change during the procedure on account of the surgeon's demand for a new team. Although personnel change is an inevitable part of surgery in order to reduce fatigue, proper and accurate sign out to the incoming team is essential to avoid unnecessary errors. In this scenario, a critical element of the procedure was the unlabeled specimens; therefore, this should have been communicated immediately to the new team or clarified before the personnel change.

This critical analysis demonstrates several examples of vulnerabilities within a single scenario. The means in which individuals interface with one another and the various components of the system (technology, environment, organizational conditions, and tasks) is of paramount importance to circumvent ambiguities and potential pitfalls that may lead to adverse events.

The Utility of Human Factors in Thoracic Surgery

Medical errors are inevitable, and often go unnoticed. Usually, a culmination of events align in a manner to bypass layers of safeguards that are in place, ultimately resulting in a clinically significant consequence. This is conceptualized using James Reason's "Swiss Cheese" model of accident causation [1]. A committed medical error can range from relatively benign, such as a missed dose of an antibiotic, to grave, such as an improperly connected chest tube, resulting in tension pneumothorax and death. The use of a human factors approach to pragmatically analyze human behavior and interaction within a system to reduce error has garnered significant interest within the field of thoracic surgery, particularly within the operating room. The operating room is a unique environment comprised of individuals with vastly different disciplines and training levels, constantly evolving technology, all in the context of high acuity and complex medical situations. Accordingly, it is no surprise that several studies have identified the operating room as a major contributor to adverse events within the hospital [2, 3]. This is especially true when examining human factors research and insights in the thoracic surgery operating room.

Learning from Our Mistakes

The commonly used adage, "never make the same mistake twice," is a simplified generalization of an objective of critical incident and near-miss reporting. These reporting systems have been broadly used in several high-risk fields, including aviation, nuclear plants, the chemical process industry, and, more recently, the medical field [4–6]. A fundamental component of incident reporting systems is the opportunity to trace a causal path, enabling the identification of active failures and latent conditions [7]. Identifying these vulnerabilities facilitates adverse event prevention in the future and is imperative in surgery to improve outcomes. Reason's model of accident causation distinguishes between active failures and latent conditions. Active failures are defined as errors triggered by an individual in the overall system (e.g., the surgeon, resident, anesthesiologist, scrub technologist, circulating nurse, etc.). Latent conditions are system vulnerabilities that are typically a result of poor decision-making by higher management in an organization (e.g., hospital administration, engineers of a technology, manufacturers) [7]. Examples in thoracic surgery of active failures include errors such as iatrogenic injury to life-threatening structures of the mediastinum (great vessels, pulmonary artery, or vein). Latent conditions include staff shortages, lack of investment in current technologies and safety measures, poor working conditions, overworked staff, and failure to invest in staff training.

Monitoring near misses or surgical failures has demonstrated to be fruitful in cardiac surgery. de Leval et al. retrospectively examined a cluster of failures (deaths) for a series of 104 neonates undergoing an arterial switch operation, ultimately finding causality with suboptimal surgical performance [8]. Using cumulative sum modeling, the group discovered that if a monitoring system of near misses had been in place earlier, an intervention (surgical retraining) could have been implemented and possibly prevented adverse events from occurring. In thoracic surgery, the tolerance for error is extremely low because the consequences of seemingly small errors have the potential to be grave. Thus, any means of preventing errors should be explored, and implemented into regular practice when feasible.

Based on the previously mentioned "Swiss Cheese" model of accident causation, the Human Factors Analysis and Classification System (HFACS) model specifically examines active and latent failures within four categories—unsafe acts, preconditions for unsafe acts, unsafe supervision, and organizational influences. The HFACS model provides an effective means of scientifically quantifying the interplay between human factors and error creation. ElBardissi et al. utilized an adapted version of the HFACS model and applied it to the cardiac OR [9]. Using structured interviews, the group demonstrated that active failures occurred infrequently and were often associated with underlying latent conditions. The most common active failures in the study were skill-based errors (a subcategory within the category of "unsafe acts"). A common response for the etiology of the skill-based errors was the high staff turnover in the cardiac OR, leading to the collective deterioration of the system itself. The high turnover inherently led to the recruitment of team members directly out of training. These individuals almost certainly lacked adequate experience needed for complex cardiac operations and high acuity situations. Organizational influences (latent conditions) were believed to be the culprit of the high turnover, secondary to deficiencies in resource management and organizational process. Examples included the lack of appropriate staff, lack of proper education and training of team members, and the burdensome logistical requirements of team members that often delayed OR time [9], as illustrated in the case study mentioned earlier.

Using monitoring systems to identify human factors involved in critical incidents and near misses provide invaluable opportunities for hospital administration, thoracic surgeons, and other team members to implement safeguards and improve outcomes. The most prudent and effective means of implementing positive change is typically addressing latent conditions that may elicit active failures.

Multidisciplinary Team and Communication

The specialty of thoracic surgery is greatly dependent on physicians of differing specialties as well as a multitude of ancillary team members of varying backgrounds, each playing a pivotal role in the care of a surgical patient (Fig. 22.2). Confounding the team dynamics include the various number of individuals that fill each role and high turnover within the field of thoracic surgery, making it near impossible to use the exact same combination of team members for every surgical case [9]. This presents an actionable opportunity from a systems standpoint (hospital administration), as maintaining surgical team consistency has proven to reduce operative time, likelihood of prolonged hospital stay, and reduce readmission rates [10, 11].

To the layman, it is instinctual to identify a single person to blame for an error. On the contrary, an adverse event can rarely be traced to a single individual, outside of blatant negligence or malicious intent. More often, an adverse event is a result of the organization predisposing a team to human error and/or failures made by the team itself. As mentioned in the cardiac chapter, Wiegmann et al. applied a human factors methodology to study surgical errors and their association with flow disruptions in cardiac surgery, ultimately discovering that the strongest predictors of committing

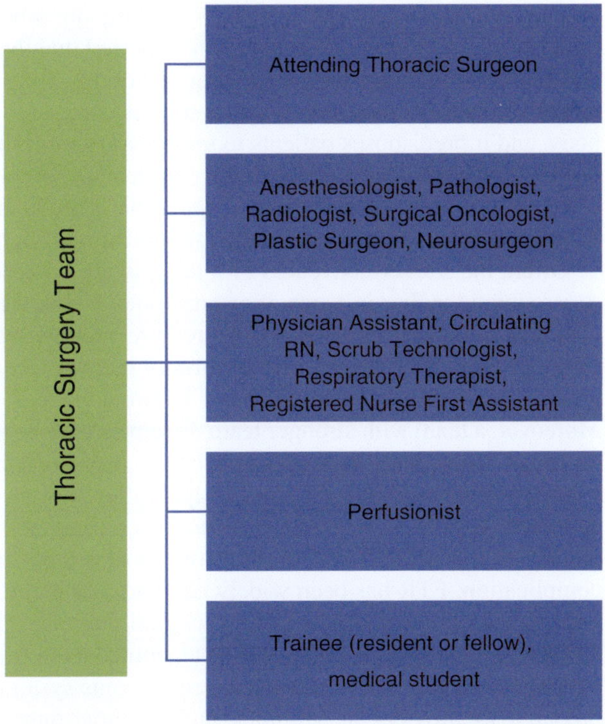

Fig. 22.2 Illustration of the possible multidisciplinary team members associated with the care of a thoracic surgery patient

an error were teamwork-related failures [11]. The specific team problems included issues related to team communication and familiarity with one another. A prospective human factors study of cardiac surgical cases revealed that teams composed of members who were familiar with the operating surgeon had significantly fewer adverse events and teamwork-related failures in comparison to those working with an unfamiliar surgeon [12]. This same study offered several interventions to improve teamwork and communication, including preoperative briefing, surgical team restructuring (promoting team familiarity), standardized intraoperative communication, postoperative debriefing, and human error training.

Communication failures are multifactorial, and often a result of environmental interference or an error in the delivery or interpretation of a message [12]. Environmental interferences, or general noise, is very common in the OR and can stem from the commonly played ambient music, nonessential communication, simultaneous communication, and equipment alerts. Given the numerous multidisciplinary team members within the OR, a standardized means of communication that avoids vague or confusing messages is critical. Closed-loop communication methods can be helpful, particularly between surgeon, anesthesiologist, and perfusionist, who have direct control of a thoracic patient's physiology and cardiovascular dynamics in the OR. A recent study identified communication failures between thoracic surgeons and anesthesiologists, resulting in foreign body entrapment (FBE)—typically, suction catheter, endotracheal tube, nasogastric tube, bronchial blocker, or temperature probe [13]. Of the surgeons who had experienced complications during pulmonary resection, 45% reported that the FBE event occurred due to ineffective communication: not asking the foreign body to be removed. This type of error can lead to increased operative time and complexity in removing the foreign body, and it predisposes patients to unnecessary morbidity. The physiologic insults on the cardiovascular and respiratory system during a thoracic surgical case can often be life threatening and thus require the surgeon and anesthesiologist to work in tandem. Effective and constant communication is paramount.

Often, the true effectiveness of a team is measured during near-miss and high-stress situations. For instance, if an anastomotic leak were to occur after an esophagectomy, this complication would require compensation by the surgical team. Compensation is described as "the form of recovery from error, where a strategy to remedy a situation is implemented before negative consequences occur" [14]. Moreover, a team with stronger team dynamics may be more effective in countering an error. Their cumulative experience may be associated with enhanced problem-solving skills, improved diagnostic capabilities, and more efficient team communication skills [14]. An indirect measure of compensation is a metric referred to as "failure to rescue" (FTR)—the inability to save a patient from death after a major complication. FTR has been widely adopted as a metric of hospital quality, and its importance has been highlighted in surgical outcomes, including those undergoing an esophagectomy [15, 16]. Silber et al. coined the term FTR as a measure of organizational and team experience, suggesting some systems or hospitals may be better prepared to provide the complex and resource-intensive care needed to rescue patients after a complication [17]. Organizational characteristics associated with adverse events include the hierarchical structure of surgical teams, high workload, overconfidence, and poor inter-professional communication [18–20]. A few of the aforementioned items may be addressed through administrative changes and team training sessions. Promoting team skills through standardized training sessions have shown to be a durable means of avoiding adverse events in high-volume thoracic surgery centers [21]. Team training sessions can underscore methodologies to conduct standardized preoperative briefing and debriefings, effective communication strategies (i.e., closed-loop communication, SBAR [situation, background, assessment, recommendation]), and situational awareness to limit flow disruptions.

Technology

The field of thoracic surgery has rapidly adopted several technologies in an effort to reduce the surgical impact on a patient and improve clinical outcomes. Despite the advantages, it is important to note that new technology can be as disruptive as it is advantageous during the learning curve and potentially beyond. For instance, the robotic platform has quickly gained significant interest from many thoracic surgeons and has changed the paradigm of minimally invasive surgery, offering a quicker learning curve to general thoracic cases than the traditional video-assisted thoracoscopic surgery (VATS) approach. However, utilizing the robotic platform introduces a new element to the system and can lead to flow disruptions, resulting in adverse events. Flow disruptions are defined as "deviations from the natural progression of an operation thereby potentially compromising safety or efficiency" [22]. Catchpole et al. utilized a human factors approach to evaluate the safety and efficiency of robotic surgery in a variety of specialties including cardiac surgery. The authors identified approximately ten flow disruptions per hour in operating rooms utilizing the robotic platform [23]. These disruptions were predominantly secondary to issues in communication, coordination, equipment, and training problems. The flow disruption rate varied by surgeon experience. Furthermore, an accumulation of flow disruptions has been associated with longer operative times, technical errors, delayed recognition of a major deterioration in a patient's condition, and omission of critical surgical steps [14, 23, 24].

As previously mentioned, surgical and team experience are imperative, particularly during complex cases, which often require intraoperative decision-making. Adding new technology such as the robotic platform will undoubtedly increase opportunities for errors during the learning curve. Despite the mandatory formal training required by all institutions, it is important to recognize that simulations cannot replace intraoperative experience. Thus, training within the OR under experienced teachers is instrumental, and during this training period, a thoughtful plan must be in place to minimize workflow disturbances and optimize patient safety. Dedicated robotic surgery teams have been suggested as a solution to mitigate the learning curve. Though this may shorten the onboarding period for the ancillary surgical staff, it may be problematic in the rare instances in which a complex case can lead to unforeseen conversion from a robotic case to an open one. If the robotic team is not experienced in open thoracic surgery, measures should be in place to address this scenario quickly and not allow patient safety to be compromised.

These challenges should not dissuade one from embracing innovative technology. Aside from the potential to enhance patient care, adopting new technology may also offer an opportunity for the working unit to make organizational changes and enhance communication and efficiency overall.

Conclusion

A single event rarely incites a consequence of clinical significance; rather, it is typically a myriad of events with which humans interface with one another, the environment, and technology that result in clinical failure. Thoracic surgery is a unique specialty in which the role of human factors research has already proven to be useful and will continue to be so as this knowledge evolves and becomes mainstream. The substantial dependence on other specialties, high complexity of cases, large multidisciplinary OR teams, and the frequent need for intraoperative decisions necessitate the need for a close evaluation of human factors to optimize workflow and prevent clinically significant errors.

Lessons Learned

- Thoracic surgery is greatly dependent on a multidisciplinary team effort. Cumulative team experience and familiarity are important predictors of efficiency and safety.
- Standardized and closed-loop communication techniques are essential in thoracic surgery given the case complexity and number of individuals involved in the operating room.
- Near-miss and critical incident monitoring systems are vital tools to analyze causation. Implementation of such review processes can lead to organizational change and improve outcomes.
- Novel technology can greatly benefit patient care and should be encouraged. However, proper planning to implement the new technology requires careful review of the learning curve, individuals involved, and the entire system as a whole.

References

1. Reason J. Human error. Cambridge: Cambridge University Press; 1990.
2. Leape LL, et al. The nature of adverse events in hospitalized patients: results of the Harvard Medical Practice Study II. N Engl J Med. 1991;324(6):377–84.
3. Thomas EJ, et al. Incidence and types of adverse events and negligent care in Utah and Colorado. Med Care. 2000;38(3):261–71.
4. Van der Schaaf TW, Lucas DA, Hale AR. Near miss reporting as a safety tool. Oxford, Butterworth-Heinemann; 2013.
5. Barach P, Small SD. Reporting and preventing medical mishaps: lessons from non-medical near miss reporting systems. BMJ. 2000;320(7237):759–63.
6. Van der Schaaf TW. Near miss reporting in the chemical process industry: An overview. Microelectronics Reliability. 1995;35(9–10):1233–43.
7. Carthey J, de Leval MR, Reason JT. The human factor in cardiac surgery: errors and near misses in a high technology medical domain. Ann Thorac Surg. 2001;72(1):300–5.
8. De Leval MR, et al. Analysis of a cluster of surgical failures: application to a series of neonatal arterial switch operations. J Thorac Cardiovasc Surg. 1994;107(3):914–24.
9. ElBardissi AW, et al. Application of the human factors analysis and classification system methodology to the cardiovascular surgery operating room. Ann Thorac Surg. 2007;83(4):1412–9.
10. Xiao Y, et al. Team consistency and occurrences of prolonged operative time, prolonged hospital stay, and hospital readmission: a retrospective analysis. World J Surg. 2015;39(4):890–6.
11. Wiegmann DA, et al. Disruptions in surgical flow and their relationship to surgical errors: an exploratory investigation. Surgery. 2007;142(5):658–65.
12. ElBardissi AW, et al. Identifying methods to improve heart surgery: an operative approach and strategy for implementation on an organizational level. Eur J Cardiothorac Surg. 2008;34(5):1027–33.
13. Schuenemeyer J, et al. Foreign body entrapment during thoracic surgery—time for closed loop communication. Eur J Cardiothorac Surg. 2017;51(5):852–5.
14. de Leval MR, et al. Human factors and cardiac surgery: a multicenter study. J Thorac Cardiovasc Surg. 2000;119(4):661–72.
15. Silber JH, et al. Failure-to-rescue: comparing definitions to measure quality of care. Med Care. 2007;45(10):918–25.

16. Liou DZ, et al. Predictors of failure to rescue after esophagectomy. Ann Thorac Surg. 2018;105(3):871–8.
17. Silber JH, et al. Hospital and patient characteristics associated with death after surgery: a study of adverse occurrence and failure to rescue. Med Care. 1992;30(7):615–29.
18. Johnston MJ, et al. A systematic review to identify the factors that affect failure to rescue and escalation of care in surgery. Surgery. 2015;157(4):752–63.
19. Donohue LA, Endacott R. Track, trigger and teamwork: communication of deterioration in acute medical and surgical wards. Intensive Crit Care Nurs. 2010;26(1):10–7.
20. Clancy CM. Care transitions: a threat and an opportunity for patient safety. Am J Med Qual. 2006;21(6):415–7.
21. Nurok M, et al. A novel method for reproducibly measuring the effects of interventions to improve emotional climate, indices of team skills and communication, and threat to patient outcome in a high-volume thoracic surgery center. Arch Surg. 2010;145(5):489–95.
22. Cohen T, et al. Identifying workflow disruptions in the cardiovascular operating room. Anaesthesia. 2016;71(8):948–54.
23. Catchpole K, et al. Safety, efficiency and learning curves in robotic surgery: a human factors analysis. Surg Endosc. 2016;30(9):3749–61.
24. Catchpole KR, et al. Improving patient safety by identifying latent failures in successful operations. Surgery. 2007;142(1):102–10.

The Application of Human Factors Research to Improve Urological Care

23

Falisha F. Kanji, Hanson Zhao, and Jennifer T. Anger

What Is Urology?

Urology is a surgical specialty, which involves treating patients with benign and malignant diseases of the male and female urinary tracts and the male reproductive organs. These organs include the kidney, ureter, bladder, prostate, urethra, pelvic floor muscles, penis, and testicles. There are several subspecialties within urology, including urologic oncology, infertility and andrology, stone disease, female urology/female pelvic medicine, neuro-urology, pediatric urology, reconstructive urology, renal transplantation, and minimally invasive surgery. Urologists perform a wide range of procedures, including vasectomies and cystoscopies, endoscopic treatments of kidney stones and bladder tumors, and robotic surgeries to remove prostate cancer and kidney masses.

Case

A 70-year-old man was admitted to the floor after an uneventful hemicolectomy. He had a history of lower urinary tract symptoms from benign prostatic hypertrophy that had been controlled with the alpha blocker tamsulosin. This medication had not

F. F. Kanji
Department of Surgery, Cedars-Sinai Medical Center, Los Angeles, CA, USA
e-mail: Falisha.Kanji@cshs.org

H. Zhao
Department of Urology, Cedars-Sinai Medical Center, Los Angeles, CA, USA
e-mail: Hanson.Zhao@cshs.org

J. T. Anger (✉)
Department of Surgery, Division of Urology, Cedars-Sinai Medical Center, Los Angeles, CA, USA
e-mail: Jennifer.Anger@cshs.org

T. N. Cohen et al. (eds.), *Human Factors in Surgery*,
https://doi.org/10.1007/978-3-030-53127-0_23

been restarted postoperatively as the patient was kept nil per os (NPO). His foley catheter was removed the morning after surgery. The nurse that day had several other complex patients and did not realize that the patient had not voided until 8 hours after the catheter was removed. The patient did complain of some suprapubic discomfort, but this was attributed to the surgical incision. The nurse called the surgery team who was scrubbed in another case but gave a verbal order to check a bladder scan. The scanner showed that the bladder had at least 600 cc of urine. The nurse called the surgery team again. They were in a critical portion of the case and did not call back for another hour, but they ultimately instructed the nurse to replace the foley. However, despite several attempts, the nurse was unable to advance the catheter into the bladder due to the enlarged prostate. A urology consult was obtained and a Coudé catheter was finally placed, with over 1.5 liters of urine immediately drained. This occurred over 12 h after the initial catheter was removed. Due to the significant amount of bladder distension, the patient was eventually discharged home with the catheter. Because of the overdistention, he had to wait a week, rather than the usual 1–2 days, to have a voiding trial. Fortunately, he followed up with the urologist and had a successful void trial 1 week after surgery.

Human Error

The Swiss Cheese Model of Accident Causation developed by James Reason discusses the way in which errors can occur in a system, beginning with small mistakes that can ultimately lead to an accident [1]. Reason describes four layers that aim to protect any system against threats that could potentially occur. However, failures or mistakes can occur at each of these layers, representing the "holes" in the "cheese". As mistakes or failures continue to occur, the opportunity for accidents or errors increases. In the medical field, mistakes such as the one that occurred in the above-mentioned case may be prevented through interventions such as the use of checklists or implementing an additional step to rounding procedures. However, medical errors continue to occur despite such interventions. For example, in South Wales, a 70-year-old male patient was in the hospital with plans to undergo a nephrectomy. The surgeon entered information into the system about the patient from an admission slip that was incorrectly completed [2]. On the day of the surgery, the surgeons had not consulted with each other about the details of the case, and the patient's surgeon did not speak with the patient prior to the operation [2]. The patient eventually went into the operating theater for his procedure where another error was made—the patient's X-ray was placed on the X-ray light backward [2]. The surgeons conducted the procedure and removed the patient's left kidney instead of his damaged right kidney. The patient later died, and the surgeons faced criminal charges. Each of the events that occurred in this accident is a prime example of how these layers of defense in the Swiss Cheese model can be broken down with preventable mistakes. Had the surgeons consulted each other, had they given more attention to the X-ray or to the information in the patient's chart, it is possible that this fatal accident could have been avoided.

Another type of error that occurs in open surgical cases are retained foreign objects. According to a study conducted by Zejnullahu, Bicaj, Zejnullahu, and Hamza [3], it was reported that approximately 1500 surgical cases per year, in the United States, involve a retained foreign object. These incidents may cause harm to the patient and require follow-up scans and procedures to resolve the issue [3–5]. So why do these accidents occur? Consider the following example: during a robotic sacrocolpopexy, a urology fellow had prepped the patient and accidentally left a sponge in the patient's vagina while simultaneously answering questions in the operating room (OR) and completing other tasks [6]. Two months after the surgery, the patient had reported that the sponge fell out of her vagina as she was walking. Fortunately, the patient did not show any signs of infection. We sought to gain a better understanding of why foreign objects were left in the vagina at our own institution. Each of the cases was analyzed using the Human Factors Analysis and Classification System (HFACS) [6]. Skill-based errors, communication, and technology were the top three reasons as to why a foreign body was retained. In a more granular analysis, these issues were most commonly associated with inaccurate counting, forgetfulness, inadequate or ineffective communication, poor design of equipment, or usability issues.

Communication, Teamwork, and Coordination

Acute urinary retention is very common in the hospital setting, and the urology service is frequently consulted to help manage this condition. We recently reviewed 1 year of urology consults for acute urinary retention and found that average volume retained in the bladder, as measured by noninvasive bladder scanner, was 860 cc [7]. This is nearly double the average bladder capacity, which is 300–400 cc, and suggests serious delays in the diagnosis of acute urinary retention [8]. In our study, patients with overdistended bladders were almost three times more likely to fail a voiding trial in the hospital and, instead, go home with a catheter. This increases their risk of urinary tract infections and catheter discomfort. Through several human factors analyses and discussions with the nursing staff, we identified multiple areas of improvement. Voiding trials should not coincide with shift changes so that they are not forgotten in a handoff or delayed. Bladder scanners should be easily accessible at every nursing station. Hospital electronic medical records can also assist by creating an order set that links a "remove Foley" order to a "check bladder scan" order. Pro re nata (PRN) (as needed) orders to replace catheters can help avoid communication delays between nurses and physicians.

Errors in communication can occur often and can contribute to mistakes that occur in the medical field. In surgery especially, communication is of the utmost importance, as errors in communication can lead to near misses or adverse events. A study conducted by Leonard, Graham, and Bonacum [9] aimed to mitigate medical errors through the improvement of communication and teamwork among medical staff. The authors describe techniques such as checklists, team briefings, and a method known as Situation, Background, Assessment, and Recommendation

(SBAR), as effective methods to improve communication between team members. The SBAR technique enforces thorough communication between team members to ensure that information is relayed appropriately. An example of this method in urological surgery can be found below:

- *Situation:* Dr. Blue, I'm calling about Mr. Green. He has had no urine output since the surgery.
- *Background:* He is a 62-year-old male who underwent a transurethral resection of a bladder tumor. He has been in the recovery room for 3 hours and has not voided since the surgery. He is also complaining of some abdominal pain.
- *Assessment:* His abdomen feels distended. I tried to perform a bladder scan, but it was not working well.
- *Recommendation:* I need you to come see him. He may need a Foley catheter and a cystogram to make sure there is not a bladder perforation.

Surgical procedures in urology are often quite complex and require effective coordination and teamwork from members who are involved in the case. Therefore, improving communication among the surgical staff can, in turn, improve coordination and teamwork. We recently conducted a focus group to discuss methods for improvement with patient and nurse experience after a sling procedure. A group of nurses were interviewed for approximately 1 hour and were asked questions about inefficiencies during patient discharge, difficulties experienced reaching surgeons when patients are unable to void, and common questions that are asked by patients about the procedure. During this focus group discussion, it was revealed that nurses often face confusion about appropriate voiding volume, when patients can be discharged, and where to place the patient's leg bag. The underlying reason these issues may be occurring could be due to surgeon preferences and patient factors. However, effective communication between nurses and surgeons may improve postsurgical processes for the patient, nurse, and surgeon.

Usability

In today's ever-changing technological world, it is important to address the topic of usability of equipment and devices in the medical field. Anyone from the patient to the surgeon can face issues with the effective use of a tool or device. It was discussed earlier in this chapter that one of the causes of a vaginally retained foreign object was the issue of usability. Human factors assessments of usability involve understanding the ease of use associated with a particular device or tool. Consider a recent study conducted by Cohen et al. [10], which aimed to understand patient preparedness, education, device usability, and satisfaction associated with sacral neuromodulation (SNM) therapy. SNM is an effective treatment for bladder dysfunction that is not responsive to more conservative therapies. SNM typically involves a 1-week testing phase in which a permanent lead is placed into the third sacral foramen (in the buttock area) but is connected to a temporary external battery. If patients experience at least 50% improvement during the testing phase, they then undergo permanent battery implantation 1 week later. Ten patients were recruited for the first phase of the study and reported difficulty with the testing device, in that it was confusing and difficult to adjust the device settings [10]. They were also confused about how to manage the bandages covering the temporary battery. An intervention was developed to increase patient satisfaction in all areas of the process—from understanding the risks and benefits of the surgery to gaining a better understanding of the device. Patients were then recruited for the second phase of the study, post intervention, and satisfaction with device in terms of usability significantly increased [10].

Conclusion

Throughout the discussion of each of these unique cases, we recognized issues with communication, teamwork, coordination, usability, and situational awareness in urology. Taking a human factors approach to improving each of these areas can be beneficial to both the medical staff and the patient. The implementation of checklists, team briefings, and process and procedural interventions for medical staff may improve patient care and reduce the rate of errors and problems that are currently faced.

Personal Pearls

1. Errors in urological surgery can adversely impact care. Human factors methods can help prevent such errors.
2. Effective communication may improve teamwork and coordination and, in turn, play a large role in decreasing the rate of errors that may occur in urological surgery.
3. Testing and incorporating human factors interventions are a simple way to improve processes and procedures, thereby leading to better patient outcomes.

References

1. Reason J. Human error: models and management. BMJ. 2000;320(7237):768–70.
2. Dyer O. Doctors suspended for removing wrong kidney. BMJ. 2004;328(7434):246.
3. Zejnullahu VA, Besnik BX, Zejnullahu VA, Hamza AR. Retained surgical foreign bodies after surgery. Open Access Maced J Med Sci. 2017;5(1):97–100.
4. Gawande AA, Studdert DM, Orav EJ, Brennan TA, Zinner MJ. Risk factors for retained instruments and sponges after surgery. N Engl J Med. 2003;348(3):229–35.
5. Brisson P. Prevention of retained foreign objects. Bull Am Coll Surg. 2009;94(11):28–31.
6. Souders C, Cohen T, Dallas K, Cohen K, Kanji F, Stewart C, Anger JT. Vaginal retained foreign objects: applying a human factors perspective. Poster presented at: Society of Urodynamics, Female Pelvic Medicine and Urogenital Reconstruction; 2020; Scottsdale, AZ.

7. Zhao H, Chen A, Cohen TN, Anger JT. High rates of unrecognized bladder overdistention among in-hospital patients with acute urinary retention: a quality problem. Urol Pract. 2019;6(6):377–8.
8. Lukacz ES, Sampselle C, Gray M, Macdiarmid S, Rosenberg M, Ellsworth P, Palmer MH. A health bladder: a consensus statement. Int J Clin Pract. 2011;65(10):1026–36.
9. Leonard M, Graham S, Bonacum D. The human factor: the critical importance of effective teamwork and communication in providing safe care. Qual Saf Health Care. 2004;13:85–90.
10. Cohen T, Burton C, Cohen K, Ackerman AL, Eilber K, Anger J. Using human factors approach to develop interventions aimed at improving patient experience with sacral neuromodulation. Poster presented at: Society of Urodynamics, Female Pelvic Medicine and Urogenital Reconstruction; 2020; Scottsdale, AZ.

Vascular Surgery: Acute Aortic Catastrophes

24

Jake F. Hemingway, Ali Azizzadeh,
and Benjamin W. Starnes

What is an Acute Aortic Catastrophe?

Acute aortic catastrophes, which include conditions such as ruptured abdominal aortic aneurysms (rAAA) and traumatic aortic injuries, represent life-threatening emergencies involving the aorta and require immediate surgical repair to prevent death. The care of these patients requires the coordinated efforts of a highly specialized team of surgeons, anesthesiologists, nurses, and technicians, who must work expeditiously and efficiently to achieve a favorable outcome.

Case Study

Imagine accepting the transfer of a patient with a ruptured abdominal aortic aneurysm from a small community hospital several hours from your metropolitan area. The transfer is delayed due to the lack of available transportation options, and upon arrival of the patient to your emergency department (ED) 5 hours later, his transport to the operating room is further delayed when the Emergency Medicine physician, who does not realize that the patient has already undergone complete imaging, mistakenly directs the patient to the computed tomography (CT) scanner. The patient then becomes hypotensive, with systolic blood pressures in the 60s, and he is

J. F. Hemingway (✉)
PGY-4 Integrated Vascular Surgery, University of Washington, Seattle, WA, USA
e-mail: heminj@uw.edu

A. Azizzadeh
Vascular Surgery Residency Program, Rosemont, IL, USA
e-mail: Ali.azzizadeh@cshs.org

B. W. Starnes
Department of Surgery, University of Washington School of Medicine, Seattle, WA, USA
e-mail: starnes@uw.edu

T. N. Cohen et al. (eds.), *Human Factors in Surgery*,
https://doi.org/10.1007/978-3-030-53127-0_24

aggressively resuscitated and rushed to the operating room. The patient is transferred expeditiously onto the operating table in the hybrid operating room; however, establishing adequate access and placing a left radial arterial line causes further delays, and upon inducing general anesthesia, the patient loses pulses. Chest compressions are started but must be interrupted intermittently to tuck the patient's arms, prep, and drape. Although the hybrid room is stocked with all of the necessary equipment in the room, the circulator and scrub tech have not previously worked with the surgeon on an acute aortic emergency. Although an access needle is available, the remainder of the items must be opened sequentially as the surgeon requests them, and ultimately the patient expires.

Now, instead, imagine the same patient scenario mentioned above within the context of well-applied protocols driving care. Upon receiving the transfer request, the receiving surgeon requests the already completed CT images to be obtained by the transfer center and notifies the emergency department of the pending transfer. Emergency medical services (EMS) personnel appropriately resuscitate the patient based on predefined blood pressure goals, and upon arrival to the emergency department, an identification band is affixed to the patient's wrist at the front desk. The patient then bypasses the emergency department and is taken directly to the operating room, which has already been prepared for the treatment of an aortic catastrophe, with all of the necessary equipment opened and ready on the back table. The patient is transferred over to the operating table, his left arm is tucked, and he is prepped and draped. The right arm is left available for anesthesia to obtain further venous access and a radial arterial line. The c-arm is brought into position from the left to allow the procedure to start. Femoral access is obtained with local anesthesia, and an aortic occlusion balloon is successfully inflated to allow for induction of general anesthesia and eventual successful graft deployment. The patient survived to discharge within 3 days.

How Can We Improve the Care of Patients with Aortic Emergencies Using Human Factors Principles?

Acute aortic catastrophes, such as ruptured abdominal aortic aneurysms or traumatic aortic injuries, represent life-threatening conditions that are almost universally fatal if not treated emergently. Historically, both conditions have been associated with high mortality rates, approaching 85% and 90% in patients with ruptured abdominal aortic aneurysms and traumatic aortic injuries, respectively, with most of these patients dying before reaching the hospital [1–3]. Even among those surviving to hospital arrival, perioperative mortality approaches 66%, and although advances in endovascular techniques and expertise are improving survival, perioperative mortality rates remain high [4–9].

Successful treatment of these acutely ill patients requires the expertise and excellent care of multiple independent members of a well-coordinated team that must simultaneously work in parallel and series to achieve a successful repair (Fig. 24.1). While the surgeon may act as the leader guiding care, the well-coordinated efforts

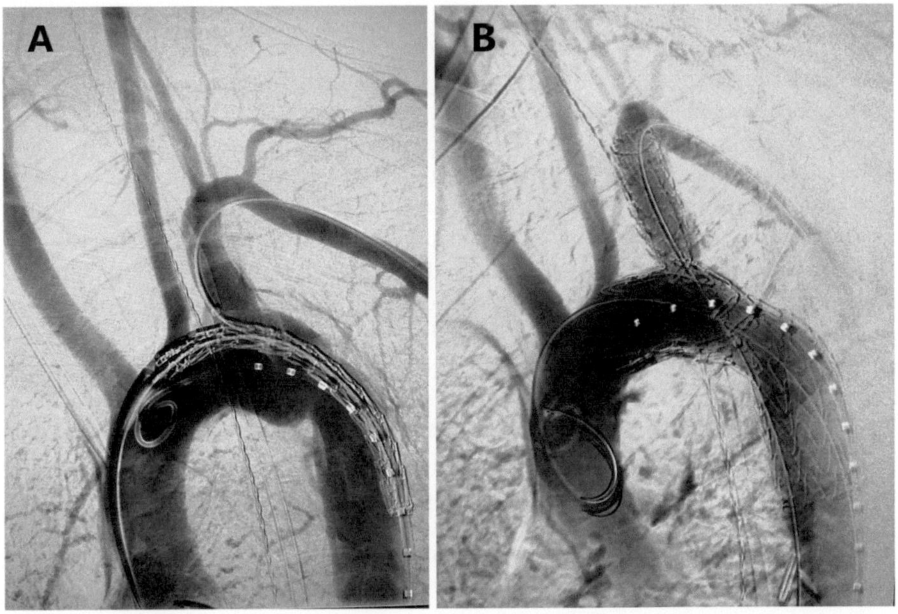

Fig. 24.1 Successful endovascular repair of a traumatic aortic injury using thoracic endovascular aortic repair. Aortic injury seen in the proximal descending thoracic aorta, immediately distal to the left subclavian origin (**a**). Successful exclusion of the injury is seen following stent graft deployment (**b**)

of anesthesia, nursing, and surgical and endovascular technicians are crucial to success. While this coordination can be achieved regularly among teams that commonly work together, these patients present at all times of the day and night, resulting in teams comprised of people who may have never worked together. It is during these cases when the lack of coordination and organization can become obvious, even with the best surgeon leaders. One cannot simultaneously do every job, and thus the surgeon relies on the initiative and anticipation of others for success. When facing aortic catastrophes, every second matters; success is dependent on organization and preparation–expectations of everyone's role must be clear.

Unlike elective cases, in which a preoperative checklist and debrief can allow the surgeon to explicitly state expectations, there is no time afforded to this preparation in emergencies, which can result in the missteps mentioned above. While an individual-focused critique of these cases will place blame upon the individual making the well-intentioned mistake, a human factors approach involves protocolizing the management for these patients, in order to create organization and coordination among team members, despite their lack of familiarity with each other or the procedure. Protocols expedite care and create care pathways that standardize the care of patients.

Expeditious care is necessary in the management of aortic emergencies. Transfer protocols ensure patients are rapidly transferred to hospitals capable of treating these emergent conditions and, when in place, ease this process. It is estimated that 24% of patients with ruptured abdominal aortic aneurysms (rAAA) are transferred, with increasing rates of transfer over time [10]. Image acquisition protocols allow transferring hospitals to rapidly upload imaging obtained prior to transfer, avoiding unnecessary reimaging upon patient arrival, and operative plans including Endovascular Aneurysm Repair (EVAR) candidacy can be determined ahead of time. Additionally, these systems ensure the availability of imaging studies to the receiving physician, as imaging is only valuable if the surgeon can see it.

In order to emergently fix a ruptured abdominal aortic aneurysm or traumatic aortic injury, one must initiate the procedure expeditiously without any unnecessary steps. In order to start the procedure, the patient must be rapidly positioned, prepped, and draped on the operating table, with the c-arm brought into position. It is important to quickly tuck the left arm at the side to allow for positioning of the c-arm. Delays introduced at any of these steps can result in death or morbidity. Previous studies have estimated that 7% of patients with rAAA die within the ED, with an additional 6% dying at the presenting hospital before undergoing treatment [11]. Although some of these deaths are likely attributable to nonoperative candidates or those in extremis, these deaths also include those patients who died awaiting treatment or transfer.

Essential to the successful creation of an acute aortic emergency protocol is determination of who should be treated, and how, such that the correct approach can be taken in treating the properly selected patients. Scoring systems exist, which help predict mortality in these conditions and should be used, as patients with 100% predicted mortality should be counseled regarding their condition, with comfort measures instituted [12]. Further, studies have shown that patients who are not candidates for EVAR but are treated with an endovascular approach do poorly, with much higher rates of morbidity and mortality [13].

Protocols also standardize the care received by patients. In acute aortic catastrophes, targeted resuscitation, permissive hypotension, and delayed institution of general anesthesia until proximal aortic control is obtained are standards that have improved survival in these patients [14, 15]. Defined blood pressure goals communicate clearly to EMS personnel how aggressive resuscitation should be. At times, these tenets run counter to the traditional training of surgeons and anesthesiologists, who are taught to protect the patient's airway before addressing circulation. Take, for example, the patient presenting with a ruptured AAA who is severely hypotensive on arrival to the OR. With systolic blood pressures in the 30s, the patient may not be protecting her airway, triggering the instinct to intubate; however, in this patient, inducing general anesthesia may result in cardiovascular collapse and death, while, instead, under no anesthesia, femoral access can be obtained and an aortic occlusion balloon placed proximally with immediate control gained and improvement in the patient's blood pressure and mentation.

Also important to treating aortic emergencies, in addition to starting the procedure, is ensuring that the correct tools are available and prepared. At our institutions, hybrid operating rooms are available for use at any time, and following the conclusion of elective cases, is specifically set up for the management of aortic

Table 24.1 Standardized aortic emergency back table setup

Access	18-gauge access needle
	1% lidocaine
Syringes	3× 20cc syringes for heparinized saline
	3× 10cc syringes for half-strength contrast
	1× 60cc syringe for aortic occlusion balloon
Wires	2× Bentson wires
	2× Glide wires
	2× stiff wires (Amplatz)
Sheaths	2× short 6 French sheaths
	2× short 11 French sheaths
	1× long 12 French sheath
Catheters	1× Kumpe catheter
	1× Vanschie 3 catheter
	1× Pigtail flush catheter
Balloon	1× CODA balloon

emergencies. This setup, listed in Table 24.1, is standardized, such that all potential on-call surgeons know exactly which tools will be immediately available at the procedure start time.

Additionally, today's information age allows for the rapid dissemination of information to anyone at the click of a mouse. While many institutions may not routinely treat aortic emergencies, treatment protocols may be created with the help of instructional videos that are readily available online. For example, our institution has created a 4-minute video, available on YouTube, on the preparation of the back table for management of an rAAA [16].

Systems and protocols make a difference in patient care, and in the treatment of aortic catastrophes, they serve as surrogates for an organized approach to improved patient care. Multiple studies have shown the improved mortality of patients presenting with rAAAs when algorithms are used (18%) versus not used (32%) [6–8]. The implementation of protocols to organize regional systems of care have allowed for the repair of 95% of patients transferred with an rAAA, with a 67% survival [17]. Although successful treatment of acute aortic catastrophes relies on an organized and well-coordinated approach, recent studies have shown that 60% of providers treating rAAA have no treatment protocols, and 70% use no transfer protocols or guidelines to expedite transfer [18]. The care of these patients can continue to improve with wider use of transfer and treatment protocols, and their dissemination represents an area for potential future improvements in care.

Lessons Learned/Personal Pearls

- To start the procedure, the patient must be rapidly transferred to the operating room, placed on the operating table, with the left arm tucked. We allow anesthesia access to the right arm for placement of IVs and monitoring lines. In the hybrid operating room, the c-arm cannot be positioned correctly, and the procedure cannot start, until the left arm is tucked, and the patient is prepped and draped. The aortic emergency cannot be addressed until the procedure starts, so every minute counts.

- Ensure that the room is set up for an aortic emergency at all times, with the correct tools available.
- Peripheral or central intravenous access is not a requirement to start the procedure as femoral venous access can be obtained quickly once an aortic occlusion balloon has been placed.

References

1. Bengtsson H, Bergqvist D. Ruptured abdominal aortic aneurysm: a population-based study. J Vasc Surg. 1993;18(1):74–80. https://doi.org/10.1067/mva.1993.42107.
2. Von Oppell UO, Dunne TT, De Groot MK, Zilla P. Traumatic aortic rupture: twenty-year meta-analysis of mortality and risk of paraplegia. Ann Thorac Surg. 1994;58(2):585–93. https://doi.org/10.1016/0003-4975(94)92270-5.
3. Attar S, Cardarelli MG, Downing SW, et al. Traumatic aortic rupture: recent outcome with regard to neurologic deficit. Ann Thorac Surg. 1999;67(4):959–64. https://doi.org/10.1016/S0003-4975(99)00174-5.
4. Visser JJ, van Sambeek MRHM, Hamza TH, Hunink MGM, Bosch JL. Ruptured abdominal aortic aneurysms: endovascular repair versus open surgery—systematic review. Radiology. 2007;245(1):122–9. https://doi.org/10.1148/radiol.2451061204.
5. Bown MJ, Sutton AJ, Bell PRF, Sayers RD. A meta-analysis of 50 years of ruptured abdominal aortic aneurysm repair. Br J Surg. 2002;89(6):714–30. https://doi.org/10.1046/j.1365-2168.2002.02122.x.
6. Larzon T, Lindgren R, Norgren L. Endovascular treatment of ruptured abdominal aortic aneurysms: a shift of the paradigm? J Endovasc Ther. 2005;12(5):548–55. https://doi.org/10.1583/04-1469.1.
7. Alsac J-M, Desgranges P, Kobeiter H, Becquemin J-P. Emergency endovascular repair for ruptured abdominal aortic aneurysms: feasibility and comparison of early results with conventional open repair. Eur J Vasc Endovasc Surg. 2005;30(6):632–9. https://doi.org/10.1016/j.ejvs.2005.06.010.
8. Moore R, Nutley M, Cina CS, Motamedi M, Faris P, Abuznadah W. Improved survival after introduction of an emergency endovascular therapy protocol for ruptured abdominal aortic aneurysms. J Vasc Surg. 2007;45(3):443–50. https://doi.org/10.1016/j.jvs.2006.11.047.
9. Mastracci TM, Garrido-Olivares L, Cinà CS, Clase CM. Endovascular repair of ruptured abdominal aortic aneurysms: a systematic review and meta-analysis. J Vasc Surg. 2008;47(1):214–221.e14. https://doi.org/10.1016/j.jvs.2007.07.052.
10. Mell MW, Wang NE, Morrison DE, Hernandez-Boussard T. Interfacility transfer and mortality for patients with ruptured abdominal aortic aneurysm. J Vasc Surg. 2014;60(3):553–7. https://doi.org/10.1016/j.jvs.2014.02.061.
11. Mell MW, Callcut RA, Bech F, et al. Predictors of emergency department death for patients presenting with ruptured abdominal aortic aneurysms. J Vasc Surg. 2012;56(3):651–5. https://doi.org/10.1016/j.jvs.2012.02.025.
12. Garland BT, Danaher PJ, Desikan S, et al. Preoperative risk score for the prediction of mortality after repair of ruptured abdominal aortic aneurysms. J Vasc Surg. 2018;68(4):991–7. https://doi.org/10.1016/j.jvs.2017.12.075.

13. Starnes BW, Garland BT, Desikan S, Tran NT, Quiroga E, Singh N. VESS26. EVAR candidacy impacts 30-day mortality for REVAR but not for open repair of ruptured abdominal aortic aneurysms. J Vasc Surg. 2014;59(6):15S–6S. https://doi.org/10.1016/j.jvs.2014.03.040.
14. van der Vliet JA, van Aalst DL, Schultze Kool LJ, Wever JJ, Blankensteijn JD. Hypotensive Hemostatis (permissive hypotension) for ruptured abdominal aortic aneurysm: are we really in control? Vascular. 2007;15(4):197–200. https://doi.org/10.2310/6670.2007.00028.
15. Dick F, Erdoes G, Opfermann P, Eberle B, Schmidli J, von Allmen RS. Delayed volume resuscitation during initial management of ruptured abdominal aortic aneurysm. J Vasc Surg. 2013;57(4):943–50. https://doi.org/10.1016/j.jvs.2012.09.072.
16. Starnes BW. Rupture Setup. https://youtu.be/FBtAbMQslzs. Published 2015.
17. Haveman JW, Karliczek A, Verhoeven ELG, et al. Results of streamlined regional ambulance transport and subsequent treatment of acute abdominal aortic aneurysms. Emerg Med J. 2006;23(10):807–10. https://doi.org/10.1136/emj.2006.037879.
18. Mell MW, Schneider PA, Starnes BW. Variability in transfer criteria for patients with ruptured abdominal aortic aneurysm in the western United States. J Vasc Surg. 2015;62(2):326–30. https://doi.org/10.1016/j.jvs.2015.03.032.

Part V

Conclusion

Final Thoughts

25

Tara N. Cohen, Eric J. Ley, and Bruce L. Gewertz

In Summary…

This text serves as an examination of the science of human factors and its role in improving safety, efficiency, and well-being in surgery. Our goal was to demystify human factors by providing a thorough discussion of its history and application in surgery. Moreover, experts of several surgical specialties demonstrated its value and application through the inclusion of unique and insightful surgical case studies.

Each author highlighted important lessons learned or personal pearls throughout their application of human factors in surgery. Regardless of their surgical specialty, they highlighted common themes that should be remembered and applied moving forward. This final chapter seeks to summarize those themes and discuss future directions.

Common Themes

Open Communication and Briefings

Communication was by far the most frequently cited term in our analysis of lessons learned. This is clearly demonstrated in the word cloud depicted in Fig. 25.1. Given that communication failures are reported as the most common attributable root cause in over two-thirds of all sentinel events in health care [1], it is not surprising that many authors highlighted the importance of effective communication to improve surgical processes.

Failures in communication are not reserved for health care. In fact, these breakdowns have been cited as the source of several well-known catastrophes in other

T. N. Cohen (✉) · E. J. Ley · B. L. Gewertz
Cedars-Sinai Medical Center, Los Angeles, CA, USA
e-mail: tara.cohen@cshs.org; Eric.Ley@cshs.org; Bruce.Gewertz@cshs.org

T. N. Cohen et al. (eds.), *Human Factors in Surgery*,
https://doi.org/10.1007/978-3-030-53127-0_25

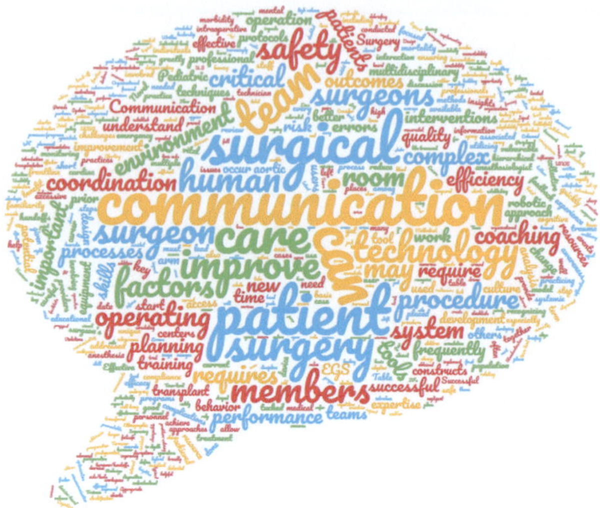

Fig. 25.1 Lessons learned word cloud. *Note a word cloud is an image composed of words used in a text or subject, in which the size of each word indicates its frequency used or importance

high-risk industries. Consider the Tenerife airport disaster of 1977 where two Boeing 747 aircraft (KLM flight 4805 and Pan Am flight 1736) collided on the runway resulting in the loss of 583 lives [2].

On March 27, 1977, a terrorist-related incident occurring at Gran Canaria Airport resulted in several flights being diverted to what is now considered Tenerife North Airport. The airport became incredibly congested and several aircraft were parked on the only taxiway (the path used for aircraft to travel on the ground, connecting them to various locations throughout an airport) available at the airport. Consequently, prior to departure or after takeoff, aircraft were required to use the runway as a taxiway by following a back-taxi procedure (the use of any portion of the runway for a taxiway where aircraft would taxi in the opposite direction from which they would land or take off). Moreover, there was reduced visibility for both the pilots and operators in the air traffic control (ATC) tower due to heavy fog on the runway.

Both aircraft (KLM flight 4805 and Pan Am flight 1736) were ready to depart from Tenerife. The ATC operators instructed the KLM pilots to taxi down the entire length of the runway and make a 180 degree turn to position for takeoff. They also asked the pilots to report back when they were ready to depart. Subsequently, the Pan Am pilots were instructed to follow the KLM aircraft down the same runway and exit by taking the third exit route available (Fig. 25.2). After getting into position, the KLM captain advanced the throttles, moving the aircraft forward. The first officer informed the captain that they had not yet received ATC clearance (the permission required to move along the runway and take off). The captain instructed the first officer to request the clearance from ATC. ATC responded with specific instructions for what to do *after* takeoff but did not include the clearance necessary for takeoff. The first officer responded to ATC saying, "we're now at takeoff". Initially, the ATC operator responded with "ok", likely because he thought the KLM pilots

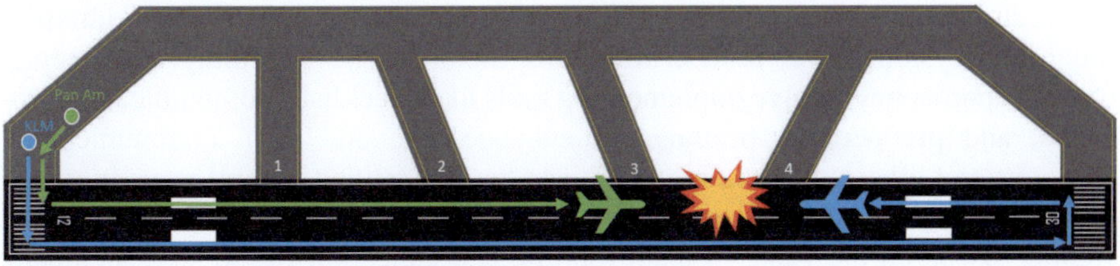

Fig. 25.2 Tenerife airport disaster (diagram)

were confirming they were *ready* for takeoff but were not yet in the process of taking off. The KLM pilots misinterpreted this response as a takeoff clearance. Immediately after saying "ok," the ATC controller communicated with KLM again, asking the pilots to "stand by for takeoff." As the ATC controller was voicing this command to the KLM pilots, the Pan Am pilots simultaneously attempted to inform the ATC controller that they were still taxiing down the runway. As a result of both communications happening at the same time, there was mutual interference on the radio frequency used to communicate. Consequently, this caused a shrill 4-second noise in the KLM cockpit, making it nearly impossible for the pilots to hear the important ATC instructions to "standby." Moreover, they missed the message from the Pan Am pilots that they were still taxiing down the runway.

The KLM pilots initiated their takeoff roll, unable to see the Pan Am plane due to the fog. The ATC operator instructed the Pan Am pilots to report when they were clear of the runway (i.e., when they exited the runway at the third exit). The Pan Am pilots confirmed these instructions. Upon hearing this communication exchange, the flight engineer on the KLM flight expressed concern about the Pan Am aircraft not being clear of the runway, but the captain indicated that the Pan Am aircraft was clear of the runway and pressed on. By the time the Pan Am pilots could see the KLM aircraft rapidly approaching, it was too late for them to maneuver the plane out of the way. On the KLM end, as soon as the pilots visualized the position of the Pan Am aircraft, they attempted to force an early takeoff in efforts to clear the plane. Unfortunately, this resulted in a catastrophic tail strike and collision into the center of the Pan Am aircraft.

As a result of this incident, the Spanish Accident Board made three recommendations: (1) placement of great emphasis on the importance of exact compliance with instructions and clearances; (2) use of standard, concise, and unequivocal aeronautical language; (3) avoid the word "takeoff" in the ATC clearance and adequate time separation between the ATC clearance and the takeoff clearance.

We tend to think of communication breakdowns as issues in the way we verbally exchange information with one another. However, especially when considering surgery, these breakdowns can manifest in several (sometimes unexpected) ways. As discussed in this text, hierarchical disparity, role conflict and ambiguity, preoperative expectations, and temporal demands can result in communication failures like mislabeling of specimens, misinterpretation of markings on a patient, and misentered information in the electronic medical records (EMR).

Because communication failures can be a consequence of individual, interpersonal, and systems-level issues, mitigating them can be incredibly challenging. Current approaches involve implementing tools like checklists, communication protocols, and preoperative briefings to enhance safe and open communication. Surgeons and other collaborating clinicians have identified several ways in which communication could be improved in the operating theatre. For example, multiple authors discussed the value of team training and education for all staff members. Others highlighted the importance of standardization and closed-loop communication and preoperative briefings to ensure effective coordination and flow prior to surgery. Finally, some argued that enhancing visualization in the OR could improve communication (e.g., developing a time-out board that everyone in the room can see, or implementing clear drapes and masks to improve information exchange between providers).

Flattening the Hierarchy

Another emerging theme of this book involves the breakdown of hierarchical boundaries and barriers. Referring to the Tenerife Disaster, accident investigators believed that the KLM captain's influence may have played a role in the catastrophe. The accident report noted that because of the captain's "great prestige," it may have been difficult for the crew to imagine that he could commit an error of this magnitude. Thus, once the captain (erroneously) claimed that the Pan Am jet was off the runway, the flight engineer and the first officer made no further objections. As a result, the Federal Aviation Administration (FAA) published the following statement in their "Lessons Learned" library (a database containing information involving aviation incidents and accidents, which aims to equip safety practitioners with knowledge to improve aviation safety): *Flight crew communications regarding airplane safety readiness should be open and effective. Each crew member must clearly give and receive communication in such a way that the flight safety decisions represent the best product of this open, two-way communication* [2].

For there to be open, two-way communication, hierarchical boundaries and barriers should be examined. The operating room (OR) tends to be very hierarchical in nature, with the surgeon traditionally at the top of the team dynamic. This dynamic is further complicated by the multi-professional nature of the OR. Because of this wide array of key players, barriers to open communication are multifactorial and can stem from a leader's interpersonal communication skills, gender differences, age differences, and lack of training in how to have open communication. Effective teamwork and communication in the OR demand the elimination of any autocracy and the support of all staff contributing to the procedure, or a flattening of the hierarchy [3].

Authors have highlighted the value of checklists, time-outs, and briefings to promote comfort in speaking up. Some have suggested that the adoption of briefing and debriefing with key members of the team will facilitate open discussions on complications or other potential challenges. Another way to break down some of these barriers may be to simply ensure that everyone knows each other's names before starting a surgical procedure.

Situational Awareness

The chapter authors consistently discussed the importance of proper coordination in the OR and often attributed successes or failures in coordination to situational awareness. Situational awareness can be simply defined as what has happened, what is happening right now, and what might happen in the future [4]. It involves having an understanding of the conditions that impact one's workflow such as the environment, timing, and the individuals involved, and it requires a continuous monitoring of a constantly evolving situation. In an ideal situation, all team members would have a shared mental model of the task at hand and how it is to be performed (in this case, surgery) [3].

Without situational awareness and shared mental models, effective team performance is nearly impossible. Let's consider basketball as an example. Coaches often spend an incredible amount of time drilling players on their ball-handling or passing skills, defensive maneuvers, and shooting abilities. However, success is also reliant upon the athletes' abilities to recognize details about their environment, the individuals they work with, and the timing of their tasks. One factor that needs to be constantly monitored is the score of the game. When there are only 30 seconds left in the game, knowing the score will impact how you respond. The team members will respond very differently if they are down four points as opposed to being up. Relatedly, team members should have a good sense of the time remaining at all points in the game. Too often players make an extra pass, eating up valuable time that could be used to attempt a shot. Paying attention to fouls can also play off during a game. Players who are cognizant of not only their own fouls but those of the other team members will be better equipped to anticipate appropriate actions at various points in the game. Finally, and perhaps most importantly, team members need to have a good understanding of their abilities as well as those of their team members. They should anticipate their team member's next moves, their positions on the court, and be knowledgeable about how they will behave. All of these skills can drastically impact the team's performance and demonstrate the importance of situational awareness.

Like basketball, team members in the operating room need to have a constant understanding of the pace of the procedure, the roles of the team members involved, and the environment they work in. They must anticipate their own needs and the needs of others. Unfortunately, training or teaching situational awareness is incredibly difficult. However, Brennan and colleagues (2020) argue that a team briefing before the start of any surgical case is the best opportunity to develop situational awareness. They also introduce SLAM, a useful mnemonic that can help to build situational awareness for individuals and the entire team. SLAM stands for *Stop*:

down tools, think through tasks and engage the brain; *Look*: is anything out of the ordinary or not quite right?; *Assess:* are you and the team prepared for the unexpected?; *Manage:* regroup, talk with the whole team, change actions as necessary [4].

Into the Future

We hope this textbook can be used as a guide for surgeons and health-care providers at any level in their training to improve their practice. We aimed to provide multidimensional human-centered insights from the viewpoint of academic surgeons and experts in human factors engineering to improve safety, efficiency and well-being in the operating room.

For those wishing to enhance their practice through the application of human factors methods, this text should serve as a foundation for understanding how this science can be applied in surgery. An ideal approach for exploring the role of human factors in surgery is to collaborate with a human factors practitioner. Unfortunately, not all medical centers have access to individuals with human factors expertise; however, there are several resources available for those interested in exploring human factors (see Table 25.1).

In conclusion, we hope this text helped to instill the idea that safety, efficiency, and well-being in surgery is impacted by more than just technical abilities of the skilled surgeon. The role of human factors in surgery cannot be understated and just may be lifesaving.

Table 25.1 Human factors resources

Resource	Description
Human Factors and Ergonomics Society (HFES) https://www.hfes.org/home	HFES is the largest scientific association for human factors/ergonomics professionals
The International Symposium on Human Factors in Healthcare	An annual symposium developed by one of HFES's largest technical groups—the healthcare group. This symposium focuses only on human factors in health care and brings together human factors experts, pharmaceutical and medical device companies, biomedical engineers, health-care providers, FDA representatives, and patient safety researchers to discuss real-world examples and experiences and find solutions for issues and challenges in health care.
Human Factors Transforming Healthcare (HFTH) Network – https://www.hfthnetwork.org	The HFTH network is a group of HF practitioners embedded in hospitals and health systems around the world. The goal of HFTH is to provide resources for HF practitioners, providers, and hospitals looking to successfully apply HF principles in their organizations.
Nielson Norman Group https://www.nngroup.com/	The Nielsen Norman Group is a user experience research and consulting firm. The founders, Jakob Nielsen and Don Norman, are known for their leadership in defining the user experience field. The website provides useful research, trainings, and suggested readings.

References

1. Commission TJ. Sentinel event statistics data: root causes by event type (2004–2014).
2. Administration FA. KLM Flight 4805 Collision with Pan Am Flight 1736 at Tenerife.
3. Wakeman D, Langham MR Jr, editors. Creating a safer operating room: groups, team dynamics and crew resource management principles: Elsevier; 2018.
4. Brennan PA, Holden C, Shaw G, Morris S, Oeppen RS. Leading article: what can we do to improve individual and team situational awareness to benefit patient safety? Br J Oral Maxillofac Surg. 2020;58(4):404–8.

Index

T. N. Cohen et al. (eds.), *Human Factors in Surgery*,
https://doi.org/10.1007/978-3-030-53127-0

MIX
Papier aus verantwortungsvollen Quellen
Paper from responsible sources
FSC® C105338

If you have any concerns about our products,
you can contact us on
ProductSafety@springernature.com

In case Publisher is established outside the EU,
the EU authorized representative is:
Springer Nature Customer Service Center GmbH
Europaplatz 3, 69115 Heidelberg, Germany

Printed by Libri Plureos GmbH
in Hamburg, Germany